# ARE YOU SUFFERING FROM THE FOLLOWING FATIGUE FACTORS?

1. After a period of rest do you still feel tired?

2. Do you have recurrent sore throats\swollen glands?

3. Do you have recurrent muscle pain?

4. Do you have difficulty thinking as clearly as in the past?

5. Do you have chronic abdominal complaints?

6. Have you had a significant decrease in sex drive?

7. Are you missing more time at work or noticing your performance decreasing?

8. Do you collapse at the end of the day or week?

9. Does intensive activity exhaust you?

## IF YOU ANSWERED YES TO ANY OF THESE QUESTIONS THEN YOU ARE HAVING SIGNIFICANT FATIGUE AND THIS BOOK IS FOR YOU!

D1247638

# AMERICA EXHAUSTED

## BREAKTHROUGH TREATMENTS OF FATIGUE AND CHRONIC FATIGUE SYNDROME

# Edward J. Conley, D.O.

Assistant Clinical Professor of Medicine
Michigan State University
College of Osteopathic Medicine
Board Certified Family Practice Physician
American Osteopathic College of Family Practice

Vitality Press
Flint, Michigan

# AMERICA EXHAUSTED
Breakthrough Treatments of Fatigue and Chronic Fatigue Syndrome

A Vitality Press Book

All Rights Reserved

Library of Congress Cataloging-in-Publication Data

Conley, Edward J.
America exhausted-breakthrough treatments of fatigue and chronic fatigue syndrome/ by Edward J. Conley

Includes bibliographical references and index.
ISBN 0-9652544-02 : $14.95
1. Severe fatigue. 2. Chronic fatigue syndrome (CFS). 3. Breakthrough treatments of fatigue. 4. Conventional medical treatments. 5. Alternative therapies. 6. Self-help guidelines. I. Title

CIP 96-060868

10 9 8 7 6 5 4 3 2 1

Printed in the United States by
Vitality Press Inc.
G3494 Beecher Road
Flint, MI 48532

# AMERICA EXHAUSTED

# Breakthrough Treatments of Fatigue and Chronic Fatigue Syndrome

To Edward P. Conley whose commitment to education has been an inspiration and in loving memory of Rita Fitzgerald Conley in which this publication fulfills her prophesy.

Also a special thanks to the staff of the Fatigue Clinic of Michigan without whose help this book would not have been possible.

# Table of Contents

# Introduction

This book will be one of the most important investments you will ever make. For the cost of two movie tickets, you will learn how to improve your energy and therefore change your life. Even if you do not have severe fatigue or chronic fatigue syndrome, the information in this book will improve the quality of your life and <u>may</u> help you to prevent serious illness in the future. If you are one of the estimated 10 million people with chronic fatigue syndrome, reading this book is an absolute must. It is vital that you understand why you are tired and what can be done to improve your vitality. Many of you, when you have sought medical attention, were told that nothing is wrong, that it is all in your head, or if you were lucky enough to have a physician that believed you, you were told that there were no treatments for your problems. <u>Nothing could be further from the truth.</u> First of all, let me state plainly that fatigue and chronic fatigue syndrome are real and serious medical conditions. They destroy lives and take the fun out of living. How do I know this? I have seen thousands of people just like you who over the last 10 years have told me their stories. People who are having problems at work, some of whom are unable to work at all. Many are failing in their interpersonal relationships and behind the eight ball in their financial matters. Most are depressed in their outlook because they have been told there is nothing that can be done. All of these things have happened because of fatigue and chronic fatigue syndrome. The good thing, however, is that <u>these</u> people have received treatment and are on their way to recovering vitality in their life. They now know what you <u>must</u> learn, that severe fatigue and chronic fatigue syndrome are treatable and there is every reason to believe that you can return to a normal life. <u>If you or a loved one are fatigued or have Chronic Fatigue Syndrome (CFS/CFIDS), you owe it to yourself to read this book.</u> For the cost of a cheap meal you will change how you feel and forever change your life!

I

# INTRODUCTION FOR THOSE WHO DO NOT HAVE FATIGUE AND CHRONIC FATIGUE SYNDROME

I believe that within the next two to three generations, the United States as we know it, may cease to exist. It may still be here in form but as far as being the most prominent economic and military force in the world, it may be gone. What will bring about the destruction of the United States? Will it come through some outside enemy force or a terrorist's nuclear bomb? No, the groundwork for the destruction of the United States has already been laid. The sad thing is, it is coming about through our own hands. Through ignorance and greed, we are selling our children's and our grandchildren's future. We will deny them the opportunities that we have had; to run, work and play with vitality. How will this catastrophe come about? FATIGUE.

Fatigue is already at epidemic proportions and it will get worse with generations to come. We are poisoning our energy production systems to such a degree that eventually this will turn the United States into a society of invalids. Taking a shower and preparing some food may consume all the energy that our grandchildren will be able to muster for the day. Some people may argue, that is okay, we will use artificial intelligence and virtual reality to accomplish what we used to do by hand. However, the use of this technology still requires intelligence, and generations of the future will find their thinking processes clouded, focusing their attention will be a real problem. Why? The energy that is required to think is generated in the same way as the energy that is required for physical activity and that is made by the Krebs cycle (a.k.a. citric acid cycle). Already the enzymes that run our Krebs cycle are being poisoned, making the production of energy more difficult. Everything leads me to believe that this poisoning will continue. If this poisoning of the Krebs cycle continues, future generations will have severe blocks in the production of energy. What is damaging our Krebs cycle? Chemicals, pesticides, herbicides, stress, vitamin and mineral deficiencies and malabsorption of nutrients. All of these factors are injuring the important enzymes that are vital for our energy production (Krebs cycle). For the sake of future generations, we must start to reverse this assault on our Krebs cycle (energy production mechanism). If we do not, the consequences will be grave. Many of the chemicals we have produced in the 20th century are waging all out war on our own bodies. You and I have been told that these chemicals are safe. Some of the time we have been misled by well meaning people, however, most of the time we have been blatantly lied to by those who wish to make money. I urge each and every American to read this book to gain a basic understanding of the problems we face since many of these same factors are also causes in the epidemic of autoimmune diseases such as lupus, asthma, MS and cancer. I urge you not to wait for bureaucrats or the government to protect you, learn this information now so that you may protect yourselves and your children.

Edward J. Conley<br>
Flint, Michigan<br>
December 20, 1996

# What Causes
# Chronic Fatigue?

Many researchers have spent years and millions of dollars looking for the one virus that causes chronic fatigue. Though somewhat simplistic, the popular approach to finding a cure for any disease is to find a single cause, be it a gene, bacterium or virus. The approach makes "sense" once you know that most medical schools teach physicians-in-training that there is always one cause for a disease. The first virus scientists identified as the "probable cause" of chronic fatigue was the Epstein-Barr virus*. Thus the original name of chronic fatigue syndrome was chronic Epstein-Barr virus disease. However, it soon became apparent that there were people with chronic fatigue syndrome symptoms who either did not have Epstein-Barr virus or were infected with other viruses.

The search for a causal virus led researchers to discover several viruses that could be causing symptoms in chronic fatigue patients. These discoveries included cytomegalovirus (CMV), the herpes simplex I and herpes simplex II viruses (HSV I, HSV II), and most recently, the human herpes virus-6 (HHV-6). Our study at the Fatigue Clinic of Michigan verified the last discovery. Fifty percent of our patients with chronic fatigue syndrome have positive IgMs for HHV-6[†]. Some scientists took the one causal virus approach in another direction.

They speculated that it is not a virus that has broken the

---

* Epstein-Barr is a herpes virus that causes infectious mononucleosis and is associated with the Burkitt's lymphoma and nasopharyngeal carcinoma.

[†] IgM is a class of immunoglobins which includes antibodies that appear early in the immune response. An IgM blood test can tell whether HHV-6 is currently a problem. A separate blood test of IgG (the most common antibodies circulating in the blood) tells whether or not the patient was ever exposed to HHV-6.

immune system. The virus is just an opportunist that creates an infection when the immune system is already worn down. Rather it is the cumulative effects of exposure to chemicals, functional blocks in the Krebs Cycle, and malabsorption of vital nutrients that leaves a person a "sitting duck" by wearing down the immune system. How does this breakdown get started? For most people, it probably starts when they are babies. Usually the first substance a child becomes allergic to is cow's milk because that is one of the first foods a baby is given*. The allergy causes swelling of the small Eustachian tubes, sinus and nasal passages. This swelling leaves babies more sus-ceptible to infection, including ear infections. Babies may or may not have an actual infection when their mothers take them to a pediatri-cian, but regardless, the doctor generally places them on antibiotics. Unfortunately, an antibiotic kills everything that is susceptible to it - good and bad. So, when children receive an antibiotic for an ear infection, the good bacteria in the sinuses, bronchial tubes, vagina (if a female) and bowel also are being killed.

After multiple infections and multiple courses of antibiotics, patients may develop what doctors term "leaky gut syndrome". In this syndrome, antibiotics have so ravaged the bowel that it has de-creased amounts of normal good bacteria and increased amounts of yeast. As a result, it does not absorb nutrients properly and allows larger molecules of food into the bloodstream than the bloodstream was meant to handle. This strain on the system triggers an antibody reaction to check the irritants.

By three to five years of age, a child initially allergic to milk may become allergic to other substances, usually common foods eaten every day, such as wheat, oats, corn or eggs. Each additional allergy upsets the immune system further. At this point, the bowel has increased amounts of abnormal bacteria, less normal bacteria and more yeast than is normal. Consequently, the bowel absorbs vitamins, minerals and amino acids poorly. (See Chapter 9-Bowel).

---

* A large percentage of mothers in the United States feed their babies formula instead of breast milk. Feeding infants formula opens them up to multiple infections and may possibly contribute to their becoming sick throughout their lifetime. I know this sounds far-fetched. However, infants get antibodies and several factors from their mother's breast milk that aid in immune system function and colonization of normal bacteria in the bowel. As I will discuss in greater detail in later chapters, normal bacteria levels in the bowel are essential for digestion. The GI tract needs normal bacteria for proper absorption of vitamins, minerals and nutrients, all of which are critical for the human body to work right.

Most people do not know that we depend on normal bowel bacteria for proper digestion. If that bacteria is reduced, we become sick.

The problems that individuals with multiple allergies experienced as children compound as they enter adulthood and encounter the environmental insults all adults experience. This includes exposure to pesticides, chemicals and stress. These people have weakened immune systems from the multiple courses of antibiotics they've taken over the years to fight infections. The enzyme systems of people, who have this condition, will eventually slow down. This is because their bodies aren't absorbing sufficient quantities of the nutrients used as cofactors for the enzymes which are necessary in the energy reactions in the body. The human body is basically a series of millions of chemical (enzymatic) reactions. Every system in the body uses chemical reactions to function normally, particularly the energy system (a.k.a: The Krebs Cycle or Citric Acid Cycle). Enzymatic reactions require vitamins, minerals and amino acids as cofactors. When the body's vitamin, mineral and amino acids levels fall, the enzyme reactions slowdown and the body's functions decline. *As your enzyme systems slow down, you slow down.*

The onset of chronic fatigue syndrome results from the progressive deterioration of enzymatic reactions rather than from an attack by a single virus. Occasionally we see people at our clinic who do not have a childhood history of allergies or multiple antibiotic use, but it is very rare. The typical patient has had multiple courses of antibiotics, sometimes for infections, sometimes for acne. Sometimes patients did not fall ill to chronic fatigue until they received heavy doses of antibiotics for a severe infection, such as pneumonia.

Patients whose enzymatic reactions are on the decline begin to experience fatigue because their bodies aren't able to generate the energy they need to work optimally. The worst part of inadequate energy production is that the immune system doesn't have the strength to do its job. *Remember, the immune system makes it's energy from the Krebs Cycle just like all other systems!* Making matters worse, sustained exposure to chemicals and an increased yeast* burden reduce immune system function further. Patients then

* Some Japanese studies done in the 1960's showed that some strains of candida albicans (yeast) can actually produce a toxin that lowers the immune system.

are like sitting ducks: easy targets for any infection that comes along. They may reactivate a virus that is already inside them, or they may pick up a new infection.

What do I mean by reactivating a virus that's already inside them? Epstein-Barr virus and the other viruses mentioned previously are very common. We all probably have some Epstein-Barr virus, cytomegalovirus and herpes simplex virus running around in us all the time. The immune system cannot eradicate each and every one of those viruses, but it can keep them under control. It's a little bit like an army trying to eradicate each and every soldier in an opposing army to be victorious. Unless the army is willing to wipe out the entire population of the opposing army's country, it's impossible to ensure the complete annihilation of the army. To be victorious, an army only needs to go in, defeat the other army, get things under control, and not worry about killing each and every opposing soldier.

The immune system acts like any well-executed army that maintains, and when necessary regains control of, a healthy environment for the body.

The immune system is extremely busy. It has to kill about two hundred cancers a day. That's right. We all develop around two hundred cancers a day, and if our immune system is strong, it kills two hundred a day. The immune system must also fight off numerous other organisms. There are millions of viruses always living in us. We have parasites wandering in and out of the body. We have bacteria and small bacterial infections. These organisms are just a few that the immune system is responsible for controlling.

Generally, the immune system is able to control the Epstein-Barr virus (as well as other organisms) which enters the body. The system kills the virus as fast as it reproduces and, therefore, the virus stays like a smoldering fire in the forest that really doesn't cause any harm unless conditions change which allow it to spread. Once the immune system function begins to slow down, Epstein-Barr viruses are not held in check. (Remember, viruses reproduce every hour. In the time it will take you to read this chapter, you will probably have two or three generations of viruses reproduce inside you). Since viruses, like all living things, reproduce exponentially, they can gain huge numbers when the immune system is not doing its job properly. The rapidly replicating viruses lead to a build up of numbers and eventually symptoms. This is what doctors call a reactivation phe-nomenon. Often, the reactivation phenomenon chronic fatigue pa-tients experience involves Epstein-Barr virus or the other viruses of the herpes family discussed in this chapter. When we talk about herpes viruses many people automatically think of genital herpes (HSVII); however there are seven members of this family including EBV and CMV. These viruses cause totally different problems other than genital herpes.

Commonly, when someone contracts an acute Epstein-Barr virus infection, their doctor says they have mononucleosis (mono). Acute mono causes swelling of the lymph glands, sore throat, sometimes swollen liver and extreme lassitude or fatigue; the patient is usually very ill. Most physicians recognize acute mono readily. Doctors used to think that mono was just something teenagers contracted. In fact, mono earned the nickname the "kissing disease" because doctors believed teenagers passed this virus back and forth by kissing each other. The symptoms of patients suffering a reactiva-tion phenomenon are usually not as severe. They don't have the full blown disease, yet they are not healthy. If they get more rest and take better care of themselves, their immune system becomes stronger and their symptoms improve somewhat. Unfortunately, if they ignore their body's needs and push themselves too hard, their immune system slows down a little bit more, the virus is able to reproduce more, and their symptoms become worse. However some people with chronic fatigue syndrome undergo the same viral reactivation scenario as people with acute mono. They endure swollen glands, sore throat, tenderness of the liver or spleen and severe fatigue. Also, sometimes people with chronic fatigue have several of the laboratory changes associated with mononucleosis; for example, positive Epstein-Barr/cytomegalovirus titers and a lowering of the white blood cell count.

What happens to the immune system in chronic fatigue syndrome? Ordinarily, the difficulty with the immune system is not a problem of limited immune cell numbers, but with how those cells actually move through the body. Immune cells (the white blood cells) must be able to move freely through the body to get at infection wherever it occurs. Usually, the cells stay in the bloodstream until an infection crops up, then they slip through the walls of the blood

5

vessels into the area where there is infection and bring the invading organisms under control. In chronic fatigue syndrome patients, the immune cells move sluggishly. Tests confirm this problem. The number of immune cells look normal on lab work, but on function studies to determine their mobility, they are not moving well. Their poor mobility may be caused by a lack of fuel due to the slow down of the enzymatic reactions. Unless the chronic fatigue patient receives active treatment of the functional blocks that decrease energy generation and get sufficient rest, their immune system will stay sluggish. Since sluggish immune cells cannot kill viruses as quickly as they reproduce, the viruses replicate to the point where the reactivation phenomenon occurs and the cycle of sore throat, swollen glands, liver tenderness and fatigue goes on.

# How Do You Know If You Have Chronic Fatigue?

Probably the best indicator that you have a problem with chronic fatigue is the fact that you are reading this book. Whether or not you fit the Center for Disease Control's criteria for chronic fatigue syndrome doesn't really matter. The reason physicians use the CDC criteria is to help them identify those people who have chronic fatigue immune dysfunction syndrome (CFIDS) *a.k.a.* chronic fatigue syndrome (CFS). The chronic fatigue criteria also allow doctors to classify extremely ill people for disability purposes and to perform studies on the disease's course.

The Fatigue Clinic of Michigan treats patients with all types of fatigue. At least fifty percent of the patients we see for chronic fatigue do not have symptoms severe enough to be classified as chronic fatigue syndrome, *but that does not mean these people are healthy.* They are still pretty sick if they meet only some of the criteria for chronic fatigue syndrome. They just don't fit a committee's definition for chronic fatigue syndrome. So, if fatigue is preventing you from participating in activities you used to enjoy, this book will offer you guidance on how to regain your health.

# CDC CRITERIA

## FATIGUE:
SEVERE, UNEXPLAINED FATIGUE, WHICH PERSISTS OR RE-LAPSES FOR 6 MONTHS OR LONGER, IT IS NOT CAUSED BY EXERTION, OR RELIEVED BY REST; HAS AN IDENTIFIABLE ON-SET (i.e. NOT LIFELONG FATIGUE); AND RESULTS IN A SUBSTAN-TIAL REDUCTION IN PREVIOUS LEVELS OF OCCUPATIONAL, EDUCATIONAL, SOCIAL OR PERSONAL ACTIVITIES.

**FOUR OR MORE OF THE FOLLOWING SYMPTOMS, WHICH MUST HAVE PERSISTED OR RECURRED DURING SIX OR MORE CONSECUTIVE MONTHS OF ILLNESS AND MUST HAVE PREDATED THE FATIGUE:**

- SHORT-TERM MEMORY OR CONCENTRATION PROBLEMS

- SORE THROAT

- TENDER CERVICAL OR AXILLARY LYMPH NODES

- MULTI-JOINT PAIN WITHOUT JOINT SWELLING OR REDNESS

- MYALGIA (MUSCLE PAIN)

- HEADACHES OF A NEW TYPE, PATTERN OR SEVERITY

- NON-REFRESHING SLEEP

- POST-EXERTIONAL MALAISE LASTING MORE THAN 24 HOURS

## EXCLUSIONS:
PEOPLE MAY BE EXCLUDED IF THEY HAVE ANY ACTIVE MEDICAL DIAGNOSIS; A PREVIOUS NON-RESOLVED MEDICAL DIAGNOSIS; PHYSICAL FINDINGS SUGGESTING EITHER OF THE FIRST TWO; MELANCHOLIC/PSYCHOLOGICAL DEPRESSION; EATING DISOR-DERS; PSYCHOSIS; ALCOHOL/SUBSTANCE ABUSE OCCURRING WITHIN 2 YEARS BEFORE THE ONSET OF FATIGUE OR AT ANY TIME AFTERWARDS OR SEVERE OBESITY.

# 3

# Does Anybody With Chronic Fatigue Ever Get Better?

Is there really a cure for chronic fatigue? Yes! The reason I'm writing this book is to let you know that chronic fatigue and chronic fatigue syndrome are real, that there are treatments available, and that *these treatments work.* People who come to the Fatigue Clinic of Michigan do get better. The majority of our patients get fifty percent improvement or more and a large percentage have regained eighty percent or more of their normal function. In essence, they have returned to normal lives. Many are back to work and they are beginning to rebuild their lives. This recovery does not mean they can go back to their old bad habits or start burning the candle at both ends again. They must always take good care of themselves (something everyone should do anyway). They must eat right, get enough sleep and control stress. What recovery does mean is that they can participate in and enjoy life again.

Doctors traditionally have been very reluctant to say there's a cure for chronic fatigue syndrome. I think we're reluctant to discuss a cure for chronic fatigue for the same reason we're reluctant to discuss a cure for cancer. We're afraid that it might recur. For cancer patients who seek treatment early, the chances of being cured are outstanding. I have several patients who have been free of cancer now for fifteen years. Yet, neither they nor I ever talk about them being cured. Though (not believed by most physicians) it is my opinion that there is indeed a cure for chronic fatigue syndrome. This book outlines the four-fold approach to treating and curing chronic fatigue syndrome that I use with my patients. We have achieved such great success at our clinic using this protocol that I wanted to

9

share it with everyone with fatigue. How do we improve energy production within the body and thereby improve the immune system as well as all the other systems in the body? By identifying and correcting blocks in the Krebs cycle. The Krebs cycle (citric acid cycle) is the complex sequence of chemical reactions that generate energy within the body. Researchers have worked out mechanisms to identify exactly where blocks exist in the Krebs cycle and how to treat them in the immune system. Studies at the Fatigue Clinic of Michigan offer significant evidence that people with chronic fatigue have functional blocks in their Krebs cycles. These blocks affect how they generate energy. Most people think we use fat, carbohydrate and protein directly as energy. We do not. We must convert those compounds into something named ATP (adenosine triphosphate). It's this ATP that we use exclusively as energy. Without ATP we don't run. Our bodies are like cars that run on gasoline. We can't pour crude oil into the tank and expect the engine to run. The crude oil does contain the energy needed to power the car, but the car can only use the energy after the oil is converted to gas. Likewise, our bodies must convert food stuffs into ATP that fuels all of our organ and enzyme systems. If you cannot generate ATP the way you should, you're going to be fatigued. How much is someone with chronic fatigue blocking ATP production? What percentage are their functional blocks? I worked in sports medicine prior to specializing in chronic fatigue syndrome. There is an old one percent rule of thumb in sports medicine. The rule claims that if you take very good athletes and improve their Krebs cycle by one percent, you could turn them into world-class athletes. Similarly, you could take world-class athletes and if you did something that slowed down their Krebs cycle by one percent, you would turn them into "also rans". I believe that people with chronic fatigue probably have a five percent reduction in efficiency of their Krebs cycles. The reduction in people mildly affected with fatigue probably is 2-3 percent, while those people who are severely affected with chronic fatigue may be up to 10 percent. Eighty percent of our energy is used as heat. Therefore a 5 percent block in Krebs cycle function causes an effective reduction of 25 percent of the energy available for all other activities (5% of 20% = 25% reduction). Every arrow on the diagram you see represents a chemical reaction in the extraction of energy from food.

## *Stages in Extraction of Energy from Food*

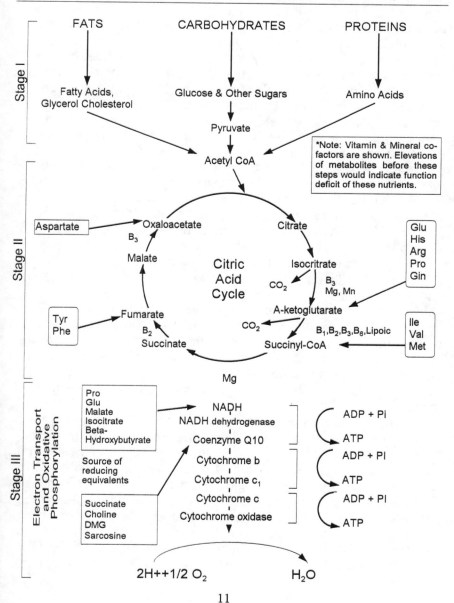

Some of the longer arrows represent multiple chemical reactions that have been simplified. Looking at the center of the diagram, you can see that vitamins, minerals and amino acids are indispensable cofactors in the citric acid cycle. One of the cycle's steps requires the cofactors of (vitamin) B3, Mg (magnesium), and Mn (manganese). Those cofactors are absolutely necessary for the energy reaction to take place at that step. When the bowel functions improperly, it does a poor job of absorbing these nutrients used as cofactors; therefore since the cofactors are low, the enzyme reactions take place ineffectively. This slow down is much like what happens on the automobile assembly line when there is a strike against a parts plant. If the strike lasts very long, it slows down the production of whatever automobile uses those parts and will eventually affect the function of the whole company. The same thing happens in the Krebs cycle. A functional block (or decrease) in one of the steps in the cycle will slow down the entire energy generation process. The process never grinds to a full halt until you die, but the slowdown affects all of your body's systems.

Most 'normal' people are able to generate energy whenever it is needed, although they may have days when they generate energy better and days when they generate it worse. People with chronic fatigue are not able to generate energy on demand as well as they should. We call this a functional block. A functional block of five percent (for example) will slow down the immune system and leave you open to viruses. It will also cause a generalized feeling of fatigue because all organs will have decreased function. That means the function of all the organs in the body may be reduced by twenty-five percent.

I often use an anecdote about my family's aging hot water heater to explain functional block to my patients. Overnight, the heater would produce a tank full of hot water. Since I was the first person up in the morning, I was able to take a nice, long hot shower, but the next person who took a shower got an ice-cold bath. Because the hot water heater was rusted and not working properly, once the hot water was drained, it couldn't recover sufficiently to meet the demand for hot water in the house the rest of the day. However, as we slept and didn't use hot water during the night, the heater could rebuild its tank of hot water—enough for my shower in the morning.

(Obviously, this disagreeable situation ended fairly quickly. We replaced the old hot water heater with a new one capable of generating energy on demand). People with chronic fatigue syndrome are like that rusted hot water heater: They cannot generate the energy they need on demand. Often my patients tell me that they have one or two "good days" during which they try to get everything they can done, followed by three or four bad days where they feel more exhausted than usual. Patients routinely tell me that if they overdo, they can almost guarantee they will throw themselves into a number of bad days. The reason for this cycle of good and bad days is that it takes a while for patients with chronic fatigue to build up their hot water tanks, so to speak. After they burn their reserves of ATP, they are not able to generate enough ATP on demand to meet their energy needs. Therefore, they feel fatigued and have to rest. (The following chapters describe how we at the Chronic Fatigue Clinic of Michigan go about improving as much as possible our patients' Krebs cycles). Usually CFIDS/CFS patients then use their Anaerobic energy production system which is very inefficient and does not produce enough energy to keep up with demand.

Another aspect of a patient's health we improve is bowel function. At one time I snickered when I heard my professor declare that the bowel is the most important organ in the body. My response wasn't any different from that of most people. Attaching importance to the bowel is a strange notion for Americans who traditionally have thought of the bowel as being almost comic. Talk about the bowel usually produces embarrassment and/or laughter. This awkwardness persists even though we constantly see advertisements for constipation and diarrhea remedies that make us more aware of bowel ailments. I don't snicker about the bowel anymore. The longer I work with chronic fatigue patients, the more I know the declaration about the bowel's importance is true. There is no improvement in chronic fatigue syndrome patients until their bowel function improves. Why is that? Because, except for oxygen, everything we need to sustain growth, repair vital processes and to produce energy must come in through the bowel. We tend to think of other organs, such as the brain, heart or liver, as being more important than the bowel. Unless the bowel absorbs food properly, the organs we consider more important won't have the substances essential for energy production and their function will be reduced.

5000 years ago the ancient Chinese said that death begins in the bowel, and they were right. The bowel is our main interface with the world around us; we are no better than our bowel absorption. We have seen over two thousand patients at our clinic with fatigue and chronic fatigue syndrome, the vast majority of whom have abnormal bowel function. Most of them have bloating, diarrhea, constipation, abnormal bowel gas, (flatus, which is rectal gas), belching and/or abdominal pain. Occasionally, there are patients who do not have any of those symptoms, but when we run tests we routinely find that their bowel function is poor.

We must distinguish here between bowel function and bowel structure. Gastroenterologists (bowel specialists) examine bowel structure by scope, barium enema or upper gastrointestinal (GI) test. They check the colon and the upper abdominal tract to determine if there is inflammation, cancer or polyps, but they are unable to determine if the bowel is actually functioning correctly. Gastro-enterologists tend to go on the mistaken assumption that if the bowel looks all right then it is functioning normally, and that is absolutely wrong! At the Fatigue Clinic of Michigan we do complete digestive evaluations on our patients to determine how their bowel is functioning. These evaluations routinely find a variety of problems: not enough normal bacteria, too much abnormal bacteria, overgrowth of yeast or fungus, parasitic infections, inadequate acid production and poor absorption of certain fatty acids just to name a few. The long and short of it is, with almost all people with chronic fatigue, bowel function is messed up!

We work very hard to reestablish normal bowel function in our patients. They need to be able to absorb vitamins, minerals and amino acids through the bowel in order to recover and maintain good health. Most of you have never thought of it this way, but the bowel is an ecosystem. A change in any portion of that ecosystem negatively impacts the whole ecosystem. A forest, too, is an ecosystem that relies on other organisms in its environment to sustain vitality. Clear-cutting the trees in a forest negatively impacts everything in the ecosystem. It exposes soil, leaving it open to erosion; it destroys the habitat of wildlife, reducing their numbers; and it decreases the production of oxygen, affecting all living beings.

A similar sequence of events occurs in the bowel when something alters its ecosystem. Normally, good bacteria line the intestine and help protect it from infection. The good bacteria also aid in food absorption, produce certain types of vitamins, (such as vitamin K) and may produce natural antibiotics that help to ward off abnormal bacteria or fungal infections. Destroying bacteria through heavy antibiotic use negatively impacts the bowel's ecosystem by reducing the layer of protection the good bacteria provide against parasites, abnormal or pathologic bacteria and viruses. It's imperative to reestablish the bowel's normal bacteria. A sound bowel works with the immune system to ward off all of these assaults as well as absorb foodstuffs in the right proportion to keep the body in maximum health. Rehabilitation of bowel function is one of the most important treatments that we do at the Clinic and has been one of the treatments that has paid the biggest dividends. (I will discuss bowel function more in later chapters).

Another goal of therapy is to do everything we can to rebuild immune function. Better nutrition is the key to this treatment step since some substances have been shown to improve immune system function. For example, vitamin C increases lymphocyte movement. Lymphocytes are the white blood cells responsible for helping us ward off viral infections. Additionally, beta-carotene, the substance produced in dark green or dark yellow vegetables, such as green leafy vegetables and carrots, has been shown to have a dose-response curve for lymphocytes. (That means reasonable supplementation increases immune function). We use a series of vitamins, minerals and nutrients to more quickly correct immune function. Another way we attempt to restore immune function and energy production is to evaluate patients for hormonal disturbances of their DHEA, testosterone or progesterone and take corrective action as needed. There are many other therapies available. (The next chapter discusses in more detail how we go about improving immune function).

The road back to health under my treatment protocol, then, has the goals of fighting viruses, increasing energy production, improving bowel function, and restoring the immune system. A word of caution is needed at this point. You won't achieve an instant cure. Most of you have been sick for months or years, and it is going to take months or years for you to get better. Now this is not to say it's going to take months or years for you to notice improvement. Many of you will feel improvement within the first few weeks of this program. However, don't become impatient. This protocol doesn't grasp at straws to uncover your problems or give you medications to cover up your symptoms. It digs down to the root problems and tries to solve them. This takes more time and effort than covering up the problems. So, hang in there! Put yourself in the healing mode and talk positively to yourself. Slowly you'll notice you're making gradual improvement and eventually, you'll return to normal health.

# Viral Illness

Most doctors and many people feel a virus causes chronic fatigue syndrome. As we discussed in Chapter 1, physicians learn during their training that there is one cause per disease. This traditional thinking generally held true because the first diseases discovered were usually caused by one virus. The polio virus causes polio and the chicken pox virus causes chicken pox. So the thinking in the medical community has been that there must be a chronic fatigue virus that causes chronic fatigue.

The Epstein-Barr virus was the first virus believed to cause chronic fatigue since so many people who had chronic fatigue syndrome symptoms seemed to have high titers of Epstein-Barr virus. (Lab tests measure titers, or concentrations of antibodies, to determine the amount of Epstein-Barr or other viruses in the body). Researchers worked hard to find a cure for chronic Epstein-Barr virus. But just as many doctors were becoming secure that Epstein-Barr virus was indeed the problem, a monkey wrench was thrown into the works. Physicians started to see people with symptoms that appeared to be chronic fatigue syndrome, yet they were not activated with the Epstein-Barr virus. They were activated with cytomegalovirus (CMV), herpes simplex virus (HSV), herpes zoster virus (HZV), or the human herpes virus type six (HHV-6), and sometimes, no virus at all. Suddenly things did not seem to make sense anymore. How could several different viruses cause symptoms that appeared to be so similar? Many doctors who treat CFS now feel that a virus does not directly cause it. Although many researchers are still getting grants to find a causal virus, many specialists feel they will never identify a chronic fatigue syndrome virus. I call the supposition that there is only one virus per disease, the mugger theory. This theory proposes that the viruses lie in wait for you like muggers in a dark alley and then overpower you against your will. While many doctors and researchers think chronic fatigue patients are mugged, or attacked suddenly, by viruses, I think they are sitting ducks whose systems finally yield to long-term stresses. After months or years on antibiotics, and the inevitable decrease in absorption of vitamins, minerals and amino acids essential for the Krebs cycle, the production of ATP falters. With a reduction in ATP, systems don't have the energy to work efficiently - that includes all systems! The immune system requires energy because it is an active system with numerous responsibilities. Once the immune systems activity slows down, the body is exposed like a sitting duck. At this point, the health of patients rapidly degenerates, either because the viruses already in them reactivate (grow faster than the immune system can kill them) or because they catch a new virus that overwhelms them. This is usually the time people remember as the exact date they became sick with a sore throat, swollen glands, cough, congestion, fever and fatigue.

I think most people believe we catch and become ill from viruses only after we're "exposed" to them. Quite the opposite is true. We have viruses living inside us all the time. Like fires smoldering in a forest, they don't harm us as long as our immune system keeps them under control. The immune system usually can keep control over Epstein-Barr and other herpes family viruses that smolder like a fire within the body. However, change conditions and the smoldering fire will blaze. In the forest the change might be wind gusts that fan sparks onto bushes and dry grass. Soon the fire spreads to the trees, and the community has a major problem on its hands. So it is with us. When the immune system becomes sluggish, the viruses which normally smolder, blaze into a fire. These viruses now can reproduce faster than the immune system can kill them. Thus, they are able to build up the numbers to make us sick.

Under normal circumstances the immune system, which is constantly on patrol, kills viruses as quickly, or nearly as quickly, as they reproduce. Though it rarely kills each and every virus in the body, the immune system constantly gains control over viruses to maintain the body's homeostasis (balance). It also attacks other invaders that are bombarding the body. These invaders may include multiple viruses, parasites, bacteria, and cancer cells. Chronic fatigue sets in when the immune system slows down due to the burdens and stresses imposed upon it and can no longer keep up with the rate of reproduction of viruses. The viruses then produce enough numbers to make us sick.

The first condition we correct when someone visits us at the Fatigue Clinic of Michigan is viral activation. We use medications to control viruses because they quickly make the person feel better. They also afford us time to improve the person's immune system so it is able to control the viruses the way that it should. We usually use a medicine called Kutapressin™ if a person is activated with Epstein-Barr virus, cytomegalovirus, or HHV-6. Kutapressin™ is a polypeptide* that is derived from pig's liver. Though most people think of liver as having iron, this medicine has no iron in it. It is actually a protein that has antiviral activities. Originally used for shingles, physicians in the United States have prescribed Kutapressin™ for over forty years. When I give lectures, doctors who are sixty years old and older know exactly what I'm talking about when I speak of Kutapressin™. Doctors who are fifty-five and under usually don't have a clue because they've never used the medicine in their practice. That's because Kutapressin™ became obsolete in this country during the 1970s after Zovirax™ was invented (or so most physicians thought!) Physicians in Europe continued to use it, however, for treatment of mononucleosis caused by Epstein-Barr and cytomegalovirus. Some U.S. researchers discovered it being used over there for mono, brought it back to this country and investigated its ability to treat chronic fatigue syndrome. They found it was effective in some CFS cases.

The exact manner in which Kutapressin™ works is unknown. The exact molecule that is active in Kutapressin™ is unknown. It is doubtful we'll ever know exactly how Kutapressin™ works, because the manufacturer seems unwilling to expend the resources to find out the mechanism. Additionally, it is doubtful that the manufacturer will ever seek U.S. Food and Drug Administration (FDA) approval of Kutapressin™ for treatment of chronic fatigue syndrome. Manuf-

---

* Peptides or polypeptides are chains of amino acids. Longer chains form proteins, while others form hormones with physiological or antibacterial activity.

19

acturers who seek approval for a new use for a medication spend millions of dollars and years of time to get it.

Kutapressin™ is already approved by the FDA for treatment of herpes zoster virus or shingles. Quite frankly, unless the odds for a large return on investment increase, no manufacturer will ever make the commitment of resources to get FDA approval for this drug for Chronic Fatigue Syndrome.

Kutapressin™ is the principal medication we use at the Fatigue Clinic of Michigan for those people who are virally activated. It produces good results; although I must warn you, it works slowly. Unlike an antibiotic that usually 'cures' a strep throat in seven to ten days, Kutapressin™ requires a standard trial of 90 to 120 days. In addition, if it seems the treatment isn't working, we increase the daily dosage from 2cc to 4cc and extend the trial period before we consider it a failure and discontinue the medication. When I first learned about the possible benefits of Kutapressin™, I used it on all my patients with chronic fatigue syndrome. The results were moderate. About forty to fifty percent of my patients responded to it. I've changed my custom in the past few years, though. Now I only use Kutapressin™ for those people I can identify as having viral activation, and our success rate has improved dramatically.

Usually we have patients inject themselves with Kutapressin™ at home on a daily basis. They administer the injections either intramuscularly or subcutaneously. Kutapressin™ is an extremely safe and effective medication. Almost everyone can tolerate it. Having been used for more than forty years, it has a long track record and its side effects are known. The only side effect of Kutapressin™ the *Physician's Desk Reference (PDR)* lists is allergy to pork. *If you are allergic to pork, you should not try this medication or you should try it only under strict physician guidance.*

The downside to Kutapressin™ is its price. It is extremely expensive, costing around $100 a vial. Most patients go through two to three vials a month. Fortunately, many insurance companies do cover Kutapressin™ prescriptions since it is on their formulary list. I alluded to another drawback earlier. There is no oral or long-acting form of Kutapressin™, so patients must inject themselves daily or every other day. Perhaps the biggest drawback is the tendency to think Kutapressin™ alone can cure chronic fatigue. Kutapressin™

injections help reduce the amount of virus in the body, but they by no means totally eradicate the virus; and it definitely doesn't fix immune system problems. That means one of two things: patients must stay on Kutapressin™ indefinitely or expect their symptoms to return when they stop the medication. That is why the remainder of the treatment program is so important. *If patients do nothing but take Kuta-pressin™, they will get improvement, but they're dooming themselves to ultimate failure.*

Regularly, physicians trying to treat a chronic fatigue patient will call me to discuss chronic fatigue and in particular, how to go about placing their patient on Kutapressin™. I always stress to them that a complete treatment program is necessary and that Kuta-pressin™ alone will not solve the problem. This emphasis on a comprehensive treatment plan is difficult for physicians to understand because they are used to giving medications and having the medications "solve the problem". In reality, medications rarely solve the underlying problem. Usually medicines treat the symptoms rather than the actual disease process. For this reason I always recommend receiving treatment from a clinic that understands the goal is to return you to health by using a comprehensive treatment plan—not just doing battle with a virus.

Zovirax™ is another antiviral medication we use at the FCM. Developed approximately twenty years ago, it is very active against herpes simplex virus. Physicians use Zovirax™ to treat severe cases of herpes simplex type one (oral herpes) and herpes simplex type two (sexually transmitted or genital herpes) cases as well as to treat herpes zoster virus (shingles). Zovirax™ is very effective against all of those viruses, but again, like Kutapressin™, it does not eradicate each and every virus, it just helps to kill them better. The advantages of Zovirax™ include that it comes in oral (pill) form and most insurance companies reimburse its cost. Disadvantages of Zovirax™ are that it is very expensive and it is not as good at treating Epstein-Barr virus and cytomegalovirus as Kutapressin™ is, nor at treating HHV-6. Until I found out that the medication has some activity against Epstein-Barr virus and cytomegalovirus, I never understood how the patients who came to me on Zovirax™ (given to them by their family doctor) could say they had some improvement. Now I believe Zovirax™ is much better than nothing at all. Zovirax™

should be used judiciously, however. As with any medication, there is the probability that during long-term uses the viruses may slowly become resistant to the medication.

While not yet FDA approved, we should discuss Ampligen™. Ampligen™ is a medication that helps regulate the antiviral defenses in our body. At one time there was great enthusiasm in the chronic fatigue community for Ampligen™. Medical practitioners thought that Ampligen™ was a "savior" for people with chronic fatigue syndrome. However, many problems have plagued the development of Ampligen™ for the market. There are conflicting reports on how well people do while on Ampligen™ and how many side effects people experience. Also, the process of gaining FDA approval for use is a slow and costly one that could potentially run into the hundreds of millions of dollars. Even if the FDA approved Ampligen™ tomorrow, it would simply be another tool for physicians to use in virally activated patients. The same underlying conditions and the same caveat would still apply that we discussed with both Zovirax™ and Kutapressin™. No medication is going to cure you of chronic fatigue; you must correct the problem with the immune system to attain a cure. In my opinion Ampligen™ is not an alternative to improving the immune system. Like Zovirax™ and Kutapressin™, it is expensive, in addition it poses the risk of unknown side effects present with all new medications. Additionally, you must stay on it the rest of your life if you don't strengthen your immune system. If you follow the chronic fatigue treatment program outlined in this book, I don't believe you will need Ampligen™ even if it should eventually be approved for use in this country for chronic fatigue. (As of 1996 Ampligen™ appears to be stalled and it is unclear if Ampligen™ will ever be released in the U.S.) We use medications as the first step in treatment of viral illnesses in chronic fatigue syndrome, not as the sole step. As I've reiterated throughout this chapter, if all we do is treat the viral illnesses with medications, then we doom the patient to either staying on the medication forever or reverting back to their old symptomatology when they stop the medicine. It is very important that patients follow the complete treatment protocol outlined in this book. No medicine that's currently available can make chronic fatigue patients healthy, and in my opinion, there will not be a medication in the future that will make chronic fatigue patients well. We must find out why the immune system is not functioning the way it should and correct those problems.

Sometimes people have chronic fatigue syndrome but do not have any identifiable viruses. What causes this baffling situation? These people probably had viral activations in the past that wreaked havoc with their enzyme systems. The injury to their enzyme systems has not allowed them to return to normal health, especially now that their immune systems are not functioning as well as they should. You can compare what is happening in these people with what happens in a region hit by a hurricane. After the hurricane dissipates, evidence of its destructive influence remains. You can tell by looking at structures, trees and vegetation that a hurricane raged through the area, even though the source of the disaster is now gone. People entering the area later who don't know there was a hurricane might wonder how the destruction occurred. The same thing happens occasionally with CFS patients. They get an activation or acute viral infection which injures their enzyme systems and leaves them disabled - or certainly not functioning normally. You can observe the effects of the virus, but you can look all you want and not find one. The inability to spot the troublesome virus could be because the numbers of the virus are now decreased and can't be picked up by testing or because the test is for the wrong virus. (We cannot test for every known virus). Another possibility is that the virus causing problems is one that hasn't yet been identified. There are probably hundreds of viruses we catch on a routine basis that researchers have not identified. Researchers identified the HHV-6 virus only within the last few years although it's existed for millions of years. (Authors note: There is now a test available to determine if a virus is part of the problem for those CFIDS/CFS patients that do not appear to have a virus. It is called the 2' 5' A Synthetase. If it is positive then there is viral activation).

Kutapressin™, Zovirax™ and other antiviral medications are effective treatments in about seventy-five percent of the cases we see at the FCM. The medications are effective only in virally activated patients and particularly, when the identity of a virus is known. We use antiviral medicines only as a tool in treating chronic fatigue and building patients' health. Our treatment plan also works to restore our patients' enzyme systems to normal. Once their enzyme systems come back and function properly, they are able then to generate the energy needed for normal function and activity.

L-Lysine is an amino acid that has anti-herpes viral activity. For years Lysine has been known to reduce HSV-1, a.k.a. cold sores. Lysine actually slows down how HSV-1 reproduces by fitting into the wrong spot on the DNA. When the DNA strands match up to reproduce there is a snag that must be repaired. An analogy for this is a zipper with a bad tooth - when you reach that point things get fouled up forcing you to fix that tooth. The HSV-1 must remove Lysine and put the amino acid Arginine in it's place. The process slows down the reproduction rate of the virus. This translates into an advantage for you—the slower the virus reproduction rate, the less viral numbers—and since viral numbers is what causes symptoms—the less symptoms.

L-Lysine appears to have activity against all of the herpes family. That includes HSV-I, HSV-II, HZV, EBV, CMV, and possibly HHV-6 and HHV-7. Lysine in general does not have any side effects. It is a natural therapy against the herpes family. Based on the knowledge that L-Lysine helps slow down reproduction of the herpes viruses *and* does not appear to have any significant side effects we have begun recommending it to patients with chronic fatigue seen at FCM.

L-Lysine does not actually kill the Herpes Virus family it just slows down how quickly they can reproduce. Since the viruses need the Amino Acid L-Arginine to reproduce, we keep the levels of L-Arginine low and the levels of L-Lysine high.

# Improvement of the Immune System and Energy Production

In the last chapter we talked about how medications alone will not solve chronic fatigue. If you're virally activated, you can use antiviral medications that will give you some improvement. However, you will eventually face two choices. One is to leave yourself on the antiviral medicines forever; the second is to take yourself off the antiviral medications after six months or a year and see how you do. The first choice is impractical because these medications are expensive and you may live another thirty to forty years. To be on an expensive medication for forty years is not the option most people would like to pursue. The second choice is not a viable option either. Although you may feel better after taking the medicine for several months, the benefits usually diminish and disappear when you withdraw from it. That is because the same underlying factors that made you sick in the first place are still present. These factors weigh down the immune system so the Epstein-Barr virus or other viruses are eventually able to build up enough numbers to again make you ill.

I try to get patients at our clinic to picture these medications as being temporary measures. Some patients do need to be on medications such as Kutapressin™ for extended periods of time (years). However, our goal is to get them off the medications as soon as possible. The way to do that is to change how your immune systems function. How do we do that? Unfortunately, modern medicine is not an exact science (despite what doctors would like for you to believe), nor is it one which the main thrust is to produce a cure based on returning you to full health. While researchers have spent billions looking for a medication to cure AIDS, they have done very few studies on ways to improve the immune system. The reason is simple economics; the company that develops a medicine to cure AIDS stands to profit *immensely*. If a fraction of the money spent to find a drug cure for AIDS had been spent to discover how to keep people healthy and improve their immune systems (once they malfunctioned), the problem of AIDS would be solved by now. Also, physicians would have a better understanding how to enhance the immune system in other diseases (i.e. CFIDS/CFS).

We do know there are certain things that seem to improve the immune system. Considerable evidence from studies done at FCM and other clinics indicates that people with chronic fatigue have multiple vitamin, mineral and amino acid deficiencies. These deficiencies act to slow down or inhibit the function of enzymes. As a person develops vitamin, mineral and amino acid deficiencies, functional blocks occur in their enzyme systems. The functional blocks slow down the production of energy of the Krebs cycle, and when that happens, all systems that run on the energy ATP (adenosine triphosphate) slow down. This slowdown affects the immune system because the immune system must have ATP to function well.

At FCM, we believe the slowdown of the immune system is caused by the baggage your immune system is carrying. We try to reduce the load of baggage. As we stated in chapter one, the breakdown of the immune system is similar to the old story about the straw that broke the camel's back. We have no way of knowing how many straws it took to break the camel's back. All we can do is grab hold of the straws as we find them, unload them and continue to unload them until eventually the camel is able to get back on its feet. This process is what we do with your immune system. We have no way of knowing how much damaging baggage your immune system is carrying or how much work it's going to take to get your immune system operating optimally. We simply know that as we find deficiencies and other problems with your immune system, we correct them. One possible cause of immune system problems is mineral deficiencies. Studies we have done at our clinic have shown that out of a hundred chronic fatigue patients, eighty percent were significantly deficient in intracellular minerals (minerals that occur inside the cell). Almost every patient had deficiencies in magnesium and chromium. Sometimes patients have normal mineral levels in the blood plasma or serum outside their cells, but their bodies are having trouble transporting the minerals into the cells where the Krebs cycle takes place.

Let's diverge for a minute and talk more about the Krebs cycle. The Krebs cycle is a series of chemical reactions that take place within almost every cell of the body. There are a few specialized cells, such as special eye cells, red blood cells and others that do not produce their own energy, but other than those few, all cells produce energy via the Krebs cycle. This takes place in the "power plant" area of the cell called the mitochondria. The minerals, vitamins, amino acids and other materials needed for the Krebs cycle must get *inside* the cell's mitochondria. This movement is not done by chance. The minerals are taken in by an active transport system. The names of the transport systems depend on what minerals the cells are taking in. For instance, the calcium-magnesium ATP-ase pump is one of the systems that actively pumps magnesium into a cell thereby allowing the magnesium to participate in the Krebs cycle. The strange thing about this process–and the catch-22 –is that ATP runs the pump. So the less magnesium the cell takes in. the less ATP it generates, the less ATP it generates, the less magnesium it can take in. This causes a negative feedback loop. Most people think that our bodies are able to burn fat, carbohydrate and protein directly as energy. But that is not true. The body must first convert those compounds to ATP, the energy used exclusively in all processes. An analogy is that automobiles cannot be powered with raw crude oil. First the crude oil must be converted into gasoline before it can run our cars. So it is with fat, carbohydrate and protein. The Krebs cycle must convert those compounds into ATP before the body can use them. All major organs in the body run on ATP: the brain, liver, lungs and heart. We literally cannot think without ATP. Additionally, ATP is needed to pump substances into cells, pump waste products out of cells and power muscle contraction for such work as walking and lifting. Our immune system runs on ATP also.

People with chronic fatigue may feel that don't have very much ATP, but that is not the case. Most people probably only have a reduction of five percent in the amount of ATP their cells are able to generate. Nevertheless, the reduction causes considerable problems for them and can result in debilitation. At the Fatigue Clinic of Michigan, we focus intensely on the Krebs cycle. You cannot improve how your immune system functions, nor increase the amount of energy you feel without improving your Krebs cycle. Our goal is always to decrease functional blocks in the Krebs cycle, so your body can better generate energy.

When there is a problem with the immune system, it can stem from two different causes: either there are not enough immune cells or the immune cells are nor moving fast enough. In chronic fatigue, the major problem with the immune system is the latter. Most patients have enough immune cells, but the cells just are not moving quickly enough (called functional activity). Their bodies have enough killer cells to fight bacterial and viral invasions, but the cells aren't able to fight hard enough because they cannot generate sufficient energy to keep up the battle. Yet, it is somewhat more complex than that because of the load on the immune system I spoke about earlier. Exposure to toxic chemicals or vitamin, mineral and amino acid deficiencies may cause slow downs (functional blocks) in ATP manufacturing. I hate to simplify the treatment of chronic fatigue, but if I had to put into one sentence how to cure chronic fatigue syndrome, it would be this: When we solve your Krebs cycle problems, we have solved your chronic fatigue. If we can get your Krebs cycles functioning at an improved level, then your health will inevitably improve.

Well, how do we improve immune function? We begin by measuring your levels of vitamins, minerals and amino acids –the substances important in the production of energy via the Krebs cycle. We do this to discover if you have deficiencies. There are many important vitamins, but certainly the B vitamins play a very important role. The Krebs cycle shows several steps where the process uses vitamins B1, B2, B3, B5, B6 and B12. It astounds me how many patients I see with functional deficiencies in B vitamins. It's bewildering since supposedly millions of Americans have responded to the bombardment of advertisements for multivitamins and are taking them. They are also eating enriched and fortified food, such as breads and cereals.

## *Stages in Extraction of Energy from Food*

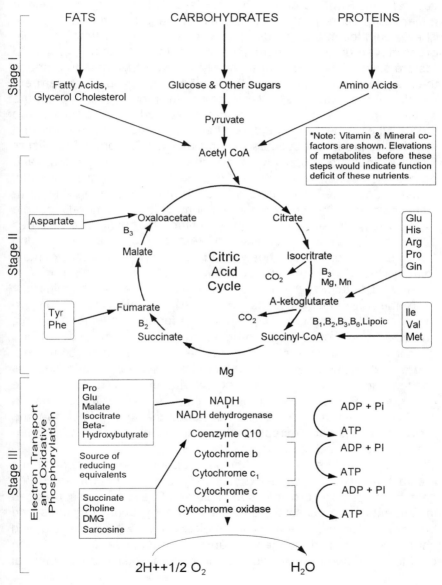

Stage I

FATS → Fatty Acids, Glycerol Cholesterol

CARBOHYDRATES → Glucose & Other Sugars → Pyruvate

PROTEINS → Amino Acids

Acetyl CoA

*Note: Vitamin & Mineral co-factors are shown. Elevations of metabolites before these steps would indicate function deficit of these nutrients.

Stage II

Aspartate → Oxaloacetate

$B_3$

Malate

Fumarate

$B_2$

Succinate

Tyr Phe

Citric Acid Cycle

Citrate

Isocitrate

$CO_2$

$B_3$ Mg, Mn

A-ketoglutarate

$CO_2$

$B_1, B_2, B_3, B_6$, Lipoic

Succinyl-CoA

Glu His Arg Pro Gln

Ile Val Met

Mg

Stage III — Electron Transport and Oxidative Phosphorylation

Pro
Glu
Malate
Isocitrate
Beta-Hydroxybutyrate

Source of reducing equivalents

Succinate
Choline
DMG
Sarcosine

NADH
NADH dehydrogenase
Coenzyme Q10
Cytochrome b
Cytochrome $c_1$
Cytochrome c
Cytochrome oxidase

ADP + Pi → ATP

ADP + PI → ATP

ADP + PI → ATP

$2H+ + 1/2\ O_2$ → $H_2O$

29

Why then are Americans, and particularly chronic fatigue patients, low in vitamins, minerals and amino acids? The reasons are several-fold. Number one is that our land is becoming depleted of minerals. In years past, farmers gave the land a chance to rebuild. They would leave their fields idle for short periods of time or would grow clover or other leguminous crops to plow under and help restore soil fertility. Nowadays, society pressures farmers to produce the maximum possible yield in the least acreage. Therefore, farmers usually till their land year after year and in a lot of cases, plant the same crop on it year in and year out. Perennially planting the same crop in the same fields depletes trace minerals from the soil and eventually, the land becomes mineral deficient. Chemical fertilizers farmers apply to crops give them the nitrogen, phosphorus and potassium needed to grow, but they don't contain trace minerals. Consequently, the foodstuffs produced from crops grown with chemical fertilizers don't contain the amount of trace minerals people need. Also, farmers used to grow maybe fifty bushels of potatoes per acre. Now, using chemical fertilizers, they grow a hundred and fifty bushels per acre. Those hundred and fifty bushels contain roughly the same amount of minerals previously found in fifty bushels of potatoes, therefore, each potato contains less minerals. From the farm, the raw foodstuffs, already depleted in minerals, go to a factory that processes them into fast foods, convenience foods, and other food products. This processing removes a great deal of the vitamin and mineral content that the raw food originally contained. The reduction in nutrients is a problem since so many foods, such as concentrated sweets, contain very few vitamins and minerals in the first place. Besides low nutritional content, some foods contain residual antibiotics and artificial hormones that may affect how the bowel functions and decreases absorption of needed vitamins, minerals and amino acids.

It cannot be overstated how important these three conditions are to fatigue in the United States. If people in the United States continue to eat food grown in soil depleted of trace minerals, reduced in nutrients by processing, and containing residual antibiotics and artificial hormones, eventually the majority of us will be afflicted with chronic fatigue. The fatigue will vary only in its severity. How much people will slow down will depend on how far their vitamin, mineral and amino acid levels have fallen and, subsequently, how far their enzyme systems (of their Krebs cycle) have reduced. It's that simple. The final reason that people with fatigue are low in essential nutrients is that people with fatigue cannot adequately absorb nutrients from the bowel. (For a complete discussion see chapter 9).

Well, how do we evaluate somebody for vitamin, mineral and amino acid deficiencies? One way is to test standard levels of vitamins, mineral and amino acids in the blood to determine whether there is a deficiency. If there is a deficiency, we assume it is at a cellular level and supplement appropriately. However, many times a person has normal plasma or serum levels of a vitamin, mineral or amino acid, but still has a cellular deficiency. This situation is a bigger problem since the vitamin or mineral is not getting into the cell where the chemical reactions take place to produce energy. Several tests can evaluate intracellular levels of vitamins and minerals. For example, the RBC mineral evaluation attempts to determine the levels of minerals within the red blood cells. If the levels of minerals are low in the red blood cells, then there is a possibility that those minerals are also low in other types of cells. To verify and remedy the deficiency, we give a clinical trial of the appropriate vitamins or minerals. (The reason why so many doctors miss these problems is that they just do the regular plasma evaluations—you must do intracellular studies. Otherwise you will miss deficiencies in the majority of people with fatigue).

Intracellular evaluations are by no means one hundred percent accurate, but they do provide some insight into what's going on in the cell. A company called Spectracell offers a study that shows promise as an evaluation tool. Called the Essential Metabolic Analysis (EMA), it is a functional evaluation that attempts to determine what vitamin or mineral is deficient (within the cell). With usual blood work a patient has their vitamin and mineral levels tested and the results are compared to the levels of thousands of individuals plotted to establish a normal range. There are several problems with this method. First, each person is an individual whose needs for vitamins and minerals are not the same as another person's. Second, the person may be treated erroneously based on a so-called normal range. For instance, the normal range for vitamin B12 in the blood is 250 to 1200. When test results come back at a level below 250, the physician suspects there is a deficiency. But what happens if the results come back at 400? Is that normal? Is more B12 needed? Could the patient benefit from more B12? The answers to these questions are unknown based solely on the traditional lab work.

Unlike most evaluations that extrapolate whether or not the person is deficient in a vitamin or mineral, based on an average range in 'normal blood', the functional evaluation attempts to establish what is needed for the individual. To do that, the EMA exposes a person's immune cells (lymphocytes) to nineteen different nutrients in individual cultures. If the lymphocytes grow better when exposed to a certain nutrient then, based on the research Spectracell has done, it means the person is deficient in that nutrient. This test gives us a way of evaluating the individual and determining individual needs. This test also gives us a way of identifying whether the patients has a functional need for further vitamin or mineral supplementation.

So there are several ways to determine whether a person is deficient in vitamins, minerals and amino acids. Each method has problems associated with it and is imperfect. However, only when the patient's physician knows which substances a person is deficient can a treatment plan be developed that resolves the functional blocks in the Krebs cycle energy production and improvement of the immune system.

# OTHER WAYS OF IMPROVING IMMUNE FUNCTION

## ANTIOXIDANTS

At FCM we employ a balanced approach to using antioxidants to improve immune function. I believe there is overwhelming evidence that antioxidants help immune function. We use a combination of B-Carotene, E, C, and Selenium along with newer antioxidants like N-acetyl-cysteine, Pycnogenol, COQ10, just to name a few. These antioxidants help prevent further cellular injury. They also help the body to detoxify many different substances including chemicals and drugs. These antioxidants help prevent injury to the immune cells themselves plus protect the Krebs cycle which is vital in making energy for the immune system.

There have been some recent studies reported where Beta Carotene did not help smokers and may even increase their risk of cancer. These studies have shown two things.

1) The foolishness of taking just one antioxidant. Nature designs us to eat a wide range of foods containing many different antioxidants all of which work together. When you use just one antioxidant you are operating in a way that nature didn't intend, therefore you will create an imbalance which usually is not productive.

2) The intellectual bankruptcy of traditional researchers who still test just one antioxidant at a time.

# 6

# Candida

In the past the medical community has generally thought candida infections were harmless—or at most a minor irritant to women with vaginal yeast. Now, there appears to be a connection between overgrowth of candida and a whole range of ailments. Candida are fungi that resemble yeasts. How do you get a candida infection? You don't really get one. Candida exist in the body all the time, especially in the mouth, vagina, and intestinal tract. The problem occurs when candida overgrow.

Very much a problem of the post-World War II baby boomers, candida overgrowth did not become an "epidemic" until the latter part of the twentieth century. It is a contributing factor of chronic fatigue and chronic fatigue syndrome (CFIDS). The reason candida over-growth is so prominent in this generation is that we are the first generation which has been exposed, on a routine basis, to the factors that cause overgrowth. Prolonged or repeated use of antibiotics, birth control pills and cortisone all have been available only since the 1940s. In addition, our diet has become much higher in simple sugar, which feed yeast, than generations before us. The stress of our modern society has also caused us to produce large amounts of cortisone within our bodies. This chronic over-production of cortisone greatly enhances yeast growth. Since the 1960's millions of American women have taken birth control pills. The average birth control user is on the drug for many years. "Candidiasis is at least doubled among birth control users"*.

Mass production of antibiotics coincided with the start of the baby boom. Considered miracle drugs, antibiotics brought under

---

* Grant, E. *The Bitter Pill. Corgi, Elm Tree/Hamish Hamilton Edition, London 1986, p.174.*

control numerous diseases caused by bacterial infections that previously killed patients. Antibiotics cured such infections as sinusitis, tuberculosis and pneumonia by killing the "bad" (disease-causing) bacteria. Unfortunately, antibiotics are not the "smart bombs of medicine": They don't target and kill only bad bacteria; they kill indiscriminately. Consequently, a course of antibiotics destroys a certain amount of "good" (or necessary) bacteria throughout the patient's body. "Virtually every antibiotic administered by mouth causes alterations in the intestinal microflora." "Pathogenic microorganisms may proliferate within the colon to fill the ecologic vacuum created by the administration of broad spectrum antibiotics[*]. Good bacteria, Lactobacillus acidophilus and bifidobacteria, produce organic acids that reduce intestinal pH and thereby inhibit the growth of acid sensitive undesirable bacteria. Lactobacillus produce lactic acid, hydrogen peroxide and possibly acetic and benzoic acids[†] Acids produced by bifidobacteria include short chain fatty acids (SCFA'S) such as acetic, propionic and butyric acids, as well as lactic and formic acids[**] the most plentiful SCFA produced by bifidobacteria is acetic acid, with a wide range of antimicrobial activity against yeasts and molds as well as bacteria[‡]. SCFA's also support normal GI function by increasing colonic blood flow, simulating pancreatic enzyme secretion, promoting sodium and water absorption and potentiating intestinal <u>mucosal</u> growth[§].

A variety of other antibacterial/anti-yeast substances have been isolated such as <u>lactocidin, lactobicillin, lactobreven</u> and acidolin[††]. These kill bacteria and yeasts directly and work as our own natural antibiotics and antifungals.

Good bacteria exist in the vagina, bowel, prostate, sinus, throat and all moist areas of the body. Lactobacillus acidophilus, lactobacillus bulgarus and other good bacteria protect the body from

[*] Simon, G.L., Gorbach, S.L. *Intestinal Flora in Health and Disease, Physiology of the Gastrointestinal Tract.* Raven Press, N.Y., pp 1361-1379, 1981.

[†] Schauss, A.G., Lactobacillus Acidophilus: *Method of Action, Clinical Application and Toxicity Data.* J Adv Med, 3 (3) pp. 163-178, 1990.

[**] Rasic, J. Lj, Kurmann, J.A. *Bifidobacteria and Their Role.* Kirkhauser Verlag, 1983.

[‡] <u>Nutritional Pearls</u> Metagenics, Vol 24, p2

[§] O'Duryn, S.T., Smith, R.J., Kripke, S.A., Settle, R.G., Rombeau, J.L., *New Fuels for the Gut, Clinical Nutrition, Enternal and Tube Feeding.* 2nd Edition WB Saunders Co.p.550, 1990.
<u>Nutritional Pearls</u> Metagenics, Vol 24,p2

[††] <u>Nutritional Pearls</u> Vol 24,pp. 17, 29-33

disease and make essential nutrients that are needed for good health. They protect us from disease by not allowing pathogens (disease-causing bacteria and yeast) to gain a foothold. The relationship between good and bad bacteria in the body is somewhat like that between grass and weeds in a well-groomed lawn. In a thick, lush lawn, the weeds find it hard to intrude. However, if harsh winter weather kills part of the lawn, next spring weeds will grow like wildfire in that area. Why? Areas left bare by winterkill give weeds access to the soil, permitting them to grow and reproduce. So it is with good bacteria in the bowel and other areas. When good bacteria are strong, bad bacteria have trouble growing and reproducing.

Previously, medical researchers thought that good bacteria were passive, i.e., they kept 'bad' bacteria from gaining a foothold—much like our lawn analogy, but recent evidence shows that good bacteria actually produce antibiotics of their own that kill pathogens. Some of these antibiotics are much stronger than penicillin. Hence, good bacteria fight pathogens two ways: through prevention and through defense.

In the United States, doctors prescribe 850 million courses of antibiotics each year. "In 1994 alone the makers of amoxicillin sold 774 tons of the antibiotic—about the same weight as two Boeing 747's. That was just the weight of the active ingredient"*. Every time you take a course of antibiotics your normal bacteria level decreases. However, antibiotics don't kill candida. Instead, as antibiotics kill off normal, essential bacteria, candida flourish. That's why you may develop diarrhea or a vaginal yeast infection from antibiotics. The more antibiotics you take, the greater potential for candida overgrowth. Why then are antibiotics over prescribed in the United States? One reason is that they are easy answers. If doctors don't know what's wrong with someone, they can prescribe an antibiotic. Another reason is that the public has come to expect antibiotics when they go see a doctor, whether the ailment warrants the treatment or not. Often, patients feel ripped off if they don't have a prescription in hand when they leave their doctor's office. They want something tangible for their money, not just sound advice.

Repeated courses of antibiotics create a vicious circle. The more antibiotics you take, the more you will have to take. Why?

* USA Today: *The Drug That Puts Kids In The Pink.* August 9,1995, pp 4D.

Because antibiotics upset the natural balance of flora in the body. This imbalance allows antibiotic resistant pathogens to grow, causing more infections and necessitating more antibiotics and so on. Additionally, candida overgrowth sometimes causes symptoms similar to infection. For example, yeast overgrowth in the sinuses may cause pressure, constant sinus drip and congestion—all of which a doctor may mistake for infection and may prescribe another antibiotic. Another serious problem is antibiotics which are fed to livestock. Farm animals receive 30 times more antibiotics than other animals. These antibiotics show up in the milk and meat that we eat[*]. As an example, 80 different antibiotics can be used to prevent udder infections in dairy cows. These antibiotics are allowed in certain concentrations in milk. A 1992 study by the Congressional General Accounting Office discovered traces of 64 antibiotics "that raise health concerns[†]."

Contributing to candida overgrowth are the stronger, wider spectrum antibiotics pharmaceutical companies constantly look for and introduce. (Wider spectrum antibiotics kill more types of bacteria, sort of like a shotgun. Unfortunately, they also hit more innocent bystanders, like a shotgun versus a rifle). There are several economic reasons why pharmaceutical companies search for wider spectrum antibiotics. 1) Old drug products go off patent after seventeen years, resulting in reduced profits for the pharmaceutical company that originally developed them. 2) New drug products are usually much more expensive for consumers, resulting in increased profits for the pharmaceutical company. 3) Old drug products are hard to market to doctors because they know about them and are less likely to talk with sales representatives about them. Consequently, doctors aren't always able to then distinguish between the products of competing pharmaceutical companies. (Drug companies don't like this). 4) Since the amount of time required to research new drug products consumes a large amount of the drug companies resources, those products must generate a big return on investment. Wider spectrum antibiotics, marketable as alternatives to older antibiotics such as penicillin and erythromycin (to which many bacteria have become resistant), fit the bill. 5) Many bacteria are now

---

[*] Nutritional Pearls: Metagenics, Vol 24, p2
[†] *ibid.*

resistant to the older antibiotics, therefore new wider spectrum ones must be used. Remember, not all bacteria are killed when an antibiotic is used. Those that are not killed are the ones that reproduce. Survival of the fittest. That's how we eventually develop antibiotic resistance—each generation is a little less sensitive to the antibiotic used until eventually the majority of the bacteria are resistant. (For a wider discussion of this problem see Chapter 12—Antibiotics).

Hormone altering drugs are the second major cause of candida overgrowth in baby boomers. Perhaps the most commonly prescribed synthetic hormone drugs are birth control pills. Widely available since the 1960s, birth control pills artificially alter a woman's hormonal cycle to prevent pregnancy. This modifying of the hormonal cycle also changes the balance of flora in the body, allowing candida to grow better. Six to ten million women in the United States have taken birth control pills, most for an average of seven years. The widespread use of birth control pills since their introduction in this country, along with the explosion in antibiotics use has fueled the incidence of yeast infections in women.

Another substance that influences the growth of candida is cortisone. Since the 1950s, doctors have prescribed this glucocorticoid as an anti-inflammatory and immunosuppressive, especially to alleviate the symptoms of rheumatoid arthritis. However, because it is a corticosteroid involved in carbohydrate, protein, and fat metabolism, when patients receive doses in amounts beyond those produced by their adrenal glands, their bodies lose their natural hormonal balance. This imbalance leaves them susceptible to candida overgrowth.

How does candida overgrowth make people sick? First, candida lowers the body's ability to absorb essential nutrients from food. To properly absorb amino acids, minerals, and vitamins in the bowel, the body needs normal levels of good bacteria. When candida is overgrown, the bowel becomes afflicted and absorption reduced. Certainly, whenever there is an overgrowth of candida, there is not enough good bacteria. Remember that good bacteria is essential to proper absorption of nutrients.

Over a period of ten or twenty years, lowered nutrient absorption pulls down a person's overall health. As your body decreases its absorption of minerals and vitamins, many of your enzymes do not work properly. Enzymes are critical to all body systems. Enzymes are essential to run all chemical reactions in the body. Therefore, changes in the way enzymes are working within the body affect the immune system, brain, liver and other organs. This reduction in enzyme function reduces the body's energy levels. Deficiencies of essential vitamins, minerals, amino acids and fatty acids particularly affect the Krebs cycle. The Krebs cycle is a sequence of chemical reactions inside the cells that are essential for the metabolism of fat, carbohydrate and proteins to energy (ATP: Adenosine Triphosphate). Dysfunction of the Krebs cycle dramatically decreases energy production and alters nearly every function in the body (since all functions of the body require energy).

Candida may also produce toxins which lower the immune function*. Although this insidious aspect of candida may sound like science fiction, it makes sense. Within nature, organisms that can survive in a hostile environment have made adaptions. Yeasts like candida are among those organisms that have evolved adaptations over millions of years. Candida albicans may have developed the ability to produce a toxin that slows down the body's natural killer cells, thereby diminishing the immune system. This adaptation is a great advantage for the yeast, but not so good for someone whose body is its host. The yeast not only survives, but thrives, while the body becomes susceptible to viral infections (because of the reduced immune function) which make the host even sicker. Worse yet, when the person visits a doctor, an antibiotic will probably be prescribed (although the illness is from a virus), decreasing good bacteria further and allowing greater yeast growth.

Thus, baby boomers and their descendants are caught in a catch-22. For some of them, the medicines considered indispensable in modern society may actually be causing them to become sick. After years of taking antibiotics or hormone altering drugs, their body's natural defense against candida has decreased. Once that defense is lowered, they become susceptible to viral infections, which in turn leads to more ailments.

To summarize: Due to the high amount of antibiotics we have been exposed to, both as medicine and in our food, the good bacteria

* Crook, William M.D. *The Yeast Connection*

in our bowel and elsewhere, has been decimated. Good bacteria is absolutely essential to our health. It is vital for absorption of nutrients from food. It prevents overgrowth of yeast, pathologic "bad" bacteria and parasites. It guards the health of all our systems that are exposed to the outside (external) environment. Many essential antibiotics are produced by good bacteria.

Mycotoxins are produced by fungi and yeasts and may have a direct toxic effect on humans. Studies have shown that many mycotoxins directly reduce immune function in humans. They are also extremely hard on liver function—the liver must detoxify these toxins, as if the liver doesn't have enough to do, except these toxins are produced inside you daily. Mycotoxins also have direct effects on the brain and nervous system. They have been studied and possibly used in the past as chemical weapons. One of the chemical weapons the U.S. was concerned about in the Gulf War was made from a mycotoxin. Mycotoxins produced in the bowel may be responsible for some of the cognitive complaints seen in patients with CFIDS/ CFS. These include memory disturbances and fuzzy thinking. They may also play a part in disruption of normal brain function such as regulation of other systems including the Endocrine system.

When good bacteria is reduced it opens the door for candida (and other yeasts) and allows it to overproduce. This over production of yeasts causes many problems.

1. Overgrowth of yeast in our bowel reduces the nutrients we absorb from our food.

2. Yeast can cause allergy to mold/yeast. The body produces antibodies to the yeast which cross-react when you are exposed to mold or yeast. This can cause a tremendous number of symptoms including: sinus congestion, asthma, muscle pain, foggy thinking and joint pain. It may also contribute to rheumatoid arthritis, lupus, M.S. and other autoimmune diseases.

3. Symptoms of burning or pain of the prostate, vagina and bladder.

4. Fatigue: resulting from the decrease in function of the Krebs cycle, reduction of our immune system with resultant viral infections, and directly from mycotoxins produced by the yeasts.

5. Bowel problems such as "Irritable Bowel Syndrome".

6. Reduction in Immune function both by reduction in Kreb Cycle function and possibly from direct toxicity to immune cells.

7. Direct low grade poisoning by Mycotoxins produced by yeasts.

# 7

# Stress

Human beings were not always as comfortable as they are now. We evolved in a time when there were great physical challenges to survival. Those challenges included getting in fights with other human beings, running away from or fighting off wild animals, and environmental stresses, such as inadequate shelter and lack of food. It was a definite survival advantage for human beings to have a system that quickly "up-regulated." An up-regulated system improved strength, the ability to fight off either another human being or an animal, or, if preferable, the ability to run away. In the process of evolution, the human body developed this system to work remarkably fast, as anyone who has a close call can attest. Within a fraction of a second of a near accident for example, the heart is pounding, the muscles are tense, and the senses are very alert. These heightened sensations are due to the stress hormones kicking in, adrenaline and other hormones that up-regulate the body's systems in the famous "fight or flight" phenomena.

The main hormone produced is epinephrine, also known as adrenaline. It is adrenaline that causes heart rate and muscle strength to increase and heightens the senses. It also helps to shunt blood away from our internal organs, making them more difficult to rupture, and pumping it into the muscles for extra energy to run or fight. Adrenaline however is also one of the strongest oxidizing agents known. Oxidation is the destructive process of nature. When a car becomes oxidized, it rusts. In human beings, oxidation causes injury to cells, collagen, DNA, enzymes and other important molecules. Most important to our discussion of fatigue, oxidation damages the enzyme systems that are vital for energy production and the normal function of nearly every system in the body. If you're being chased by a tiger, you don't worry about the oxidative damage that the adrenaline is doing to your body. You either get away from the tiger - or you won't have to worry about it! The fight or flight mechanism evolved to ensure survival, and it has definite survival benefits. Those people who had well developed fight or flight mechanisms survived better than people who didn't and were alive to reproduce. That's why everyone now has them. You can compare the boost in adrenaline your body produces in an emergency to the boost in power Indy car racers can activate by pressing the boost button in their race cars. The button is invaluable, particularly when the race is on the line and a driver must make a last pass coming in to the final turn to win the Indianapolis 500. Drivers can press the boost button to give their engine that extra spurt needed to maneuver their car around their opponent and into the winner's circle. Race drivers know, however, if they leave their finger on that button a fraction too long, the engine will blow. The same disastrous effect can happen when your body produces too much adrenaline. (Although, unlike Indy cars, we may take years to 'blow').

Meant for emergency purposes only, adrenaline is the body's boost button. The problem is, nowadays we have very few emergencies requiring an energy boost, yet adrenaline gets pumped into our system. We no longer get in fights with other people on a regular basis. We don't have to run away from or defend ourselves against wild animals. Our physical needs are generally met—we have all the food we need to eat and we live in a relatively well-controlled climate. Stresses today are much different and are long-term. However, the human body has only one mechanism for handling stress, and that is the same mechanism that our ancestors had ten thousand years ago for running away from tigers: the production of adrenaline, cortisone, and those other stress hormones. (The fight or flight response).

For the long-term stresses we face in the twentieth century, we still rely on those hormones to get us through. Whether our house is being repossessed or we're going through a divorce, we use the same hormones as our ancestors did when a tiger was chasing them. Now, granted we do not use as much hormone as quickly, but we use tremendous amounts of these hormones over a longer time. Indeed, such complicated legal and psychological issues as divorce or financial problems may last for several years. During that time, we draw on those chemicals heavily, even though this system was not meant for long-term use. Due to the long-term pumping of adrenaline into our bodies, over real or perceived threats, oxidation severely damages our enzyme systems. Our enzyme systems lose their ability to regulate energy production and control other systems. This causes another problem. The longer we rely on our adrenals to produce the chemicals we need to handle stress, the more fatigued the adrenals become, and the less adequately we're able to handle stress. What used to seem like mild stresses to us, now seem overwhelming. We start to become worn down, as our adrenals become more and more fatigued from the long term stress we place on them.

The systems our bodies use to handle stress are complex. Central to those systems are the adrenal glands, which are the size of a hickory nut. When you compare their size to that of the liver, which may weigh several pounds, it's easy to understand that the adrenals are not meant for long-term over use. The adrenals rely heavily on proper nutrition and require a significant amount of nutrients to produce hormones. They also require rest time. Good sleep and long rest periods recharge them. After an animal escapes danger in the wild, it finds safe shelter and rests. This rest allows the animal's adrenals to recover and permits down-regulation of all the stress hormones that were produced during the chase. Unfortunately, people rarely give themselves a chance to relax and recover from high levels of stress hormones. Often we go from stress to stress to stress until, for some of us, even previously pleasant activities become unbearably stressful. We've become so tense, and so stressed, that we end up hurrying for everything, and end up stressing ourselves even in times when there are no external stressors.

So, a combination of factors wear down our adrenal glands, resulting in adrenal fatigue. One factor is the effect of long-term stress itself, which, even for a person in optimum nutrition, can eventually wear them down. The second factor is poor nutrition. Most Americans have significant nutritional deficiencies that make them more vulnerable to the effects of stress, both in how they handle it and how well their adrenals are able to recover from it. Thirdly, we have very little time for rest; we do not allow our adrenals to recover adequately after we experience stress.

Stress does not necessarily have to come from outside of us, to be a physical stress. Frequently, it comes from within. It is not unusual for me to have patients at the Fatigue Clinic of Michigan who've suffered either physical, psychological, or sexual abuse as children. Most psychiatrists would say these people are fatigued because they are depressed. I have a different opinion about their condition. I know it is a physiological—and psychological—problem. When I talk with these patients about their problems, they usually reveal how much psychological stress they've placed on themselves for years, often since childhood. Whether they have done it consciously or subconsciously, they have punished themselves literally for years because of what happened to them and many have developed poor self-esteem. This internal self-punishment has put an incredible drain on their systems, wearing them down to where now they're not able to handle the external stresses in their lives either. At the Fatigue Clinic, we attempt to guide these people out of their self-punishment, so they can put their minds to rest and allow their bodies to heal. Another massive problem we now face in the U.S. are the scars on children caused by divorce. (Not to mention the scars on adults!) With nearly 50% of marriages ending in divorce, (many times these are not amicable, to say the least), the children are often caught in the middle, leaving them with long term stress and worn down adrenals. Not only the people who've suffered physical, psychological, or sexual abuse, but all of us suffer from perceived stresses or perceived dangers. Something happens (maybe not even to us) and we think of what bad thing could possibly happen to us in the future. Sometimes we dwell on the possibilities for days or weeks at a time. These thoughts of perceived danger place strain on our bodies just as much as actual danger*. As we'll talk about in another chapter, often patients end up reaching for drugs in an attempt to help them cope with the stresses or relieve some of the feelings of stress. These drugs are only a short-term "fix" and will ultimately result in the patient being further worn down and the fatigue symptoms worsening. If you took a poll today of

* Studies have shown that our bodies react nearly the same to perceived danger as to real danger.

physicians and people on the street, my bet is that most would say stress is the number one killer in the United States. I would agree. Many times when I work with patients in stop-smoking programs, the biggest factor that we must deal with, along with their nicotine addiction, is how they are going to handle stress since they use cigarettes as a crutch for stress. Similarly, in working with patients in weight loss and food management programs, I've found that many people use food as a crutch to handle stress. When they are under stress, they eat more and they eat the wrong things. (They may respond that way because of nutritional deficiencies*). Stress also affects the body's response to disease. Stress contributes to coronary artery disease. I have had several pathologists tell me that they have autopsied patients who died from a coronary myocardial infarction (heart attack) without finding a blood clot clogging the artery, although the patients may have had fifty or sixty percent occlusion of the artery. In many cases, pathologists tell me, they think stress causes the arteries to go into spasm, and it's that spasm that ultimately killed these people. Certainly, stress contributes to the development of cancer by pulling down the immune system so that the person does not kill the cancers as they develop. Remember, you develop two hundred cancers a day, and your body must kill two hundred cancers a day. If your immune system is not strong, your body cannot do this. Also as I pointed out earlier, stress causes long term production of adrenaline which results in oxidative damage to DNA, ultimately resulting in cancer.

So, stress, in my mind, is the number one killer in the United States and a major cause of fatigue in the U.S. The question we have to ask ourselves is, why are our lives so stressful? What have we done to make them so stressful? If they're not that stressful, why do we perceive them as being so stressful? Let's look at these questions one at a time. No one would argue that the United States has changed dramatically over the last generation. In the 1940s and 1950s, life was lived at a slower pace. Families ate meals at home. There was usually one member of the household who took care of

---

* We conducted a study of 99 people with CFIDS/CFS. The results showed 86% were low in the amino acid Tyrosine. Tyrosine is needed to make Epinephrine (Adrenaline). Chocolate is high in Tyrosine. Also, 56% were low in Tryptophan—Tryptophan is an essential amino acid needed to make Serotonin. Serotonin is an important brain chemical in coping with stress and preventing depression. Carbohydrates temporarily raise Serotonin levels in the brain.

the household chores and one who worked outside the home to provide an income. The foods we ate were more wholesome, less preserved, and higher in vitamins and other nutrients. There were fewer pressures coming at us. There was a general sense of prosperity, time to live life, to have a family, flourish in your job, and have the American Dream of owning your own house and car. The broadcast industry was in its infancy; advertisers had yet to develop the high pressure sales pitches they bombard us with today. By the 1990s, our life-style has changed radically. We no longer feel content with the old standard of the American Dream: an average house and car. We want the largest house, more than one car, and recreational vehicles for every member of the family*. To attain this new standard, both parents in two-parent households work, leaving the children to fend for themselves. In nearly half of the households in the United States, only one parent is present. That parent is doing two jobs; providing for the family and also trying to raise the family. This situation puts tremendous stresses on the parent and on the children. The foods we eat are low in vitamins and minerals that would help our body cope with stress. The over indulgence in processed and junk food along with the exhausting of our land has lead to food that is too low in nutrients.

There are many, many more factors which have caused our society to become so stressed. Most of them are beyond the scope of this book, but most people would agree stresses are much greater in the 1990s than they were in the 1950s. Also, few would argue that we made those stresses ourselves.

Oftentimes, our own choices, our own demands have caused us to place our health in jeopardy. We must reach a point where we ask ourselves the question, is all of this worth dying for? I routinely get asked by patients, how do we reduce our stress? People often don't see any way out. I always recommend they begin with small changes to their life-style. Small changes are much easier than large changes and usually are the ones they can live with the longest. Most of their stress would be gone if they could move to Tahiti and live a life-style of relaxation, but for most of us that's not practical.

Often times, by the time I see patients, chronic fatigue has

---

* Not to mention a vacation house, trips to Europe and our kids in the most prestigious private Universities.

47

placed a severe strain of them, both personally and professionally. They feel they are a failure personally because they are not able "to hold up their own end" in a relationship or in the family. They feel that they're not being the spouse or parent that they should be since they are not able to do the things they would like to do around the home. I always urge them to simplify their lives as much as possible by changing their goals, especially regarding possessions. I advise them to evaluate what their true goals in life are, what their aspirations are, and what is worthwhile to pursue. By evaluating their options, they can determine how to take control of their situation. I counsel them at length that they have to remember what a parent and spouse is. A parent is not a chauffeur and does not need to be one. Children do not necessarily need attention twenty-four hours a day, and neither does a spouse. Rather, I tell my patients to make the time spent with a spouse or children count—even if it's only a half-hour a day —by sharing news and activities with each other and focusing on what's really important and not worrying about small annoyances. I also counsel patients to start looking on the positive side even though their financial concerns may be mounting as they struggle with chronic fatigue. I remind them that they will get better and advise them that professional help is available to help them get their finances in order. If they are disabled by chronic fatigue, they may be eligible for Social Security or other government benefits or for aid from private agencies. Mainly, they need to do whatever is necessary to reduce the short-term stresses, realizing that in the future they will be more productive and able to do those things they currently are unable to do. The key to reducing stress is to figure out what is important in life and prioritize activities accordingly.

The most important thing people with chronic fatigue can do, other than seeking a professional who understands how treat chronic fatigue, is to find a place of healing and peace within themselves. I recommend my patients begin meditation, self-hypnosis, or biofeedback sessions or classes. At the Fatigue Clinic we offer classes in relaxation and breathing and self-hypnosis. I advise patients to practice these techniques daily so they learn to relax their muscles by breathing slowly and regularly from their diaphragms. Under stress, internal organs do not get the blood they need and eventually will become impaired. Ulcers, irritable bowel syndrome (with cramping and bowel spasms), Crohn's disease, ulcerative colitis or any number of problems of the internal organs may occur from this impairment. Relaxation allows blood to better enter internal organs, and it reduces muscle tone in the skeletal muscles. Muscles under stress are tense and burn tremendous amounts of energy.

Perhaps the best prescription I give my patients is the direction to find a quiet spot each day where they can be by themselves and take time to turn their minds off and allow their bodies to reach a state of relaxation, a state of healing, a state of peace. Once they learn how to relax, they do not react to stresses as strongly and thus can control their physiology better to keep the production of adrenaline to a minimum. They again begin to use adrenaline only when absolutely necessary, which is the purpose for which it was intended. For a complete discussion of a relaxation technique called autoregulation please read *The Canary and Chronic Fatigue* by Dr. Majid Ali.

## Important Points

1. Stress is extremely destructive in everyone —especially someone with fatigue.

2. The way it is destructive is by producing adrenaline which is an extremely destructive hormone. Adrenaline was developed for short -term use only —not for long-term use—which is usually how we use it today.

3. You can not control many of the things that happen to you, but you can control how you react to them. Thereby reducing stress.

4. Meditate or pray daily—this helps reduce stress and reduce the production of the destructive chemicals that accompany it. The con- stant production of theses chemicals—through stress—further in- jures the already damaged energy production system.
(The Krebs cycle).

## Stress

Stress may be the number one reason why so many people are sick in the U.S.

1. Stress is not just mental—it has definite physical ramifications and causes defined physical changes.

49

2. The body responds the same to mental and emotional stressors as it does to physical stressors.

3. The body's response is the same rather the threat is actual <u>or</u> perceived.

4. How does the body respond to stress? "The fight of flight scenario".

5. Why do we have this response? It is vital for survival—Survival of the Fittest.

   A. What happens during the fight or flight response?

      Glucogenesis: develops energy needed to fight (or run away from danger).

      Decreased blood flow to organs.
         1. An organ that is full of blood is much easier to rupture —this has obvious consequences on the survival of the being.

         2. Helps to raise blood pressure and heart rate. To fight (or run) your blood pressure needs to go up.

      Increased Catecholamines like Norepenephine helps quicken reflexes, heightens alertness, and improves strength.

      All of these responses have developed over millions of years through the process of natural selection—all aimed at one thing, <u>survival</u>. These were aimed at survival in the world as it <u>was</u> between the beginning of time and now. These adaptations were developed for a world that is much different from the one we live in today. Today's threats are from deadlines, regulations, traffic jams, lawsuits—not threats on our bodies like animal or human attack or extreme weather. Most of our threats today are mental and are prolonged.

Our survival mechanism was developed to cope with stress that lasted hours or days. In an attack by an animal or another human we either were strong enough to fight off the attacker or fast enough to get away or we were dead. In any case this lasted several minutes. Harsh weather may have lasted days or in extremes maybe weeks, but humans did not develop this stress system to be used for months or years. When we use our stress system for months or years we cause tremendous damage due to the overproduction of Adrenaline.

Our body when it is under stress will steal other hormones to make Cortisone out of them. The body sees cortisone as being the most important hormone when under stress as it helps us to survive. We developed mechanisms to make more cortisone if the body is under stress. The body does this by stealing the hormones DHEA and Progesterone from other pathways (Pregnenolone Steal Pathway). This may be one reason why if we put a woman under enough stress her menstrual periods will become abnormal or even stop— the body sees the manufacture of cortisone as the most critical thing to do*. Besides, the last thing nature wants is for the woman under stress to have a baby (remember stresses in the past meant times were not good, i.e. not enough food or harsh weather or illness). The same thing happens to a man—under stress the body steals testosterone to make cortisone out of it—that's why when under stress a man's sex drive goes down.

The other thing the body does is "steal" DHEA to make cortisone out of it. The exact functions of DHEA are poorly understood. We know that DHEA plays a function in improving immune status (animal studies indicate that DHEA has a direct stimulating effect on T-lymphocytes[†].

So what happens to us when we are under stress for months or years? Our body continues to produce cortisol which when elevated over the long term lowers our immune function. We begin to get chronic infections (like EBV, CMV, HSVI & HSVII and HHV-6) because of lower immune function. Our body becomes low in progesterone or testosterone causing menstrual abnormalities and

---

* The body "steals" pregnenolone to make cortisone, therefore less is available to make estrogen and progesterone.
[†] Daynes, R. et al 1990

loss of muscle energy and strength (fatigue). Our levels of DHEA drops causing further lowering of our immune function. We retain Na+,CO2, H2O and deplete H+, K+ and Mg+. The retention of sodium and water contribute to HYPERTENSION. In others the adrenals wear down (adrenal fatigue) causing hypotension (low blood pressure) secondary to loss of sodium and water.

So we now have a person with lower sex drive and/or menstrual abnormalities. Their immune system is down so they get infections easily, either chronic viral infections or bacterial infections which require multiple courses of antibiotics (see Candida chapter). They have a decrease in muscle strength and endurance (because of lack of DHEA and testosterone —also because of mineral loss). They have difficulty generating energy because of functional blocks in the Krebs cycle (because of mineral deficiency and also stress damage to the Krebs cycle - see chapter on Krebs cycle). They may have had multiple courses of antibiotics causing increased Candida, and therefore a decrease in absorption of nutrients in the bowel.

I hope by now you get the idea—does this sound like anyone you know? So although we see stress as this mental problem—it has definite physical ramifications. If stress is prolonged we develop serious physical problems which lead ultimately to <u>BURN OUT</u>! We have not even scratched the surface of the body processes that begin to malfunction when we are under long-term stress. Our sleep cycle becomes abnormal. This results in difficulty falling asleep or staying asleep. Stress may cause lack of normal sleep cycles—loss of REM sleep. REM sleep is where the body restores the neuro-chemicals in the brain. Without proper neurochemicals in the brain—cognitive function may slow. The decrease in brain neurochemicals also leads to depression. The causes of the sleep disturbances are numerous:

1. Hypoglycemia: (see hypoglycemia chapter) Blood sugars fluctuate at night as well as day. When the sugar drops low, the body produces catecholamines (adrenaline) to cause release of stored starch from the liver (this brings up blood sugar). The release of adrenaline however may stimulate the person and cause awakening or alterations in the sleep cycle. Hypoglycemia is caused by the wearing down of the adrenals by long term stress.

2. Abnormal Melatonin: Under stress the body reduces the production of melatonin. Melatonin is the chemical the body produces that causes us to go to sleep. The reduction in melatonin causes insomnia and abnormal stages of sleep.

3. Abnormal Adrenal Response: Elevations of cortisone at night (escape of HPA suppression). Cortisone levels should be lowest at night. This causes stimulation when it should be time for sleep.

4. Amino Acid deficiencies: Lack of certain amino acids will contribute to sleep disturbances. This is one explanation for the phenomenon in #3. The amino acid Tryptophan is needed to make Serotonin. Serotonin is important to fight depression, improve immune function and keep a normal sleep cycle. 56% of people with CFIDS are low in tryptophan (FCM clinical study); therefore, they are low in serotonin. Melatonin is important in trying to recover from chronic stress —Melatonin, among other things, improves the deep stage of sleep. As I pointed out before, deep sleep is needed to clear the brain of waste products and the replenished neurochemicals needed for proper function. The majority of patients with fatigue are probably low in melatonin. The deficiency of serotonin and melatonin may be respondsible for the abnormal changes in the sleep cycle of people with fatigue.

5. Other factors: Many other factors may play a part in disturbance of the sleep cycle such as various vitamin and mineral deficiencies. (See Chapter 8 Sleep, Chapter 10 Depression, Chapter 11 Hypoglycemia and Chapter 15 Adrenal Fatigue).

## Adrenal Cortical Adaptation to chronic stress.
## Pregnenolone "Steal" by the Cortisol Pathway

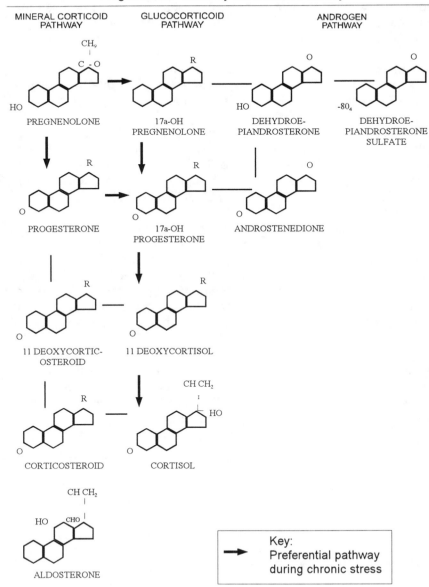

| MINERAL CORTICOID PATHWAY | GLUCOCORTICOID PATHWAY | ANDROGEN PATHWAY |
|---|---|---|

PREGNENOLONE

17a-OH PREGNENOLONE

DEHYDROE-PIANDROSTERONE

DEHYDROE-PIANDROSTERONE SULFATE

PROGESTERONE

17a-OH PROGESTERONE

ANDROSTENEDIONE

11 DEOXYCORTIC-OSTEROID

11 DEOXYCORTISOL

CORTICOSTEROID

CORTISOL

ALDOSTERONE

Key:
Preferential pathway
during chronic stress

54

# 8

# The Importance of Sleep

Sleep disturbance is a major problem for patients with chronic fatigue and chronic fatigue syndrome. Almost everyone with chronic fatigue complains of sleep disruption. The more severe their fatigue, the more severe their sleep problem, and vice versa. The disturbances become worse as their fatigue becomes worse, creating a downward spiral. Most of us pay little attention to sleep. We tend to think of sleep as a luxury and not a necessity. However, sleep is an absolute necessity. Sleep is the time when our body replenishes itself. One of the major reasons we require one-third of our day in sleep is to renew our brain neurochemicals. Without our neurochemicals, we have trouble thinking and behaving normally. Why our body requires so much sleep we don't know, but it is a well known fact that without enough sleep, our body's function slows down significantly. Some people can manage on much less sleep than others. Former President Kennedy, for instance, was known to be able to function on four hours sleep a night, while President Clinton suffices on five plus a nap. For most people, eight hours of sleep a night is considered the norm.

I see two sleep disturbance problems in my chronic fatigue patients. The first is quantity of sleep and the second is quality. Let's talk first about quantity. If you miss one hour of sleep each night, and only get seven hours of sleep instead of eight, that means you get seven fewer hours of sleep a week, or nearly one less day of sleep per week. That calculates out to a loss of twenty-eight hours of sleep a month. In a year you would lose three hundred and thirty-six hours, that equals forty two eight hour nights, or almost one-and-a half months of sleep. If you continue to lose sleep, in five years you will have missed over seven-and-a-half months of sleep, or well over one-half year of sleep. It is estimated that lack of sleep alone causes a loss in productivity of fifty billion dollars per year in the United

States. While sleep disturbances take their toll on 'normal, healthy' people, they are more harmful for those with chronic fatigue.

The problems patients with chronic fatigue have with sleep, however, go far beyond not getting to bed early enough. Their quantity of sleep becomes abnormal because they have difficulty falling to sleep, and when they do, they have difficulty staying asleep. I once tested a patient who woke up over three hundred times during the night. The patient did not realize she was waking up, but our sleep study showed she was coming out of sleep that often. With such frequent disruption of her normal sleep pattern, it was no wonder she was sick. Ninety percent of my patients tell me they have some abnormalities of sleep. The question patients usually ask me is, Doctor, how can I be so exhausted during the day, yet when I go to bed at night, I can't fall asleep for hours? How can this be? There are a number of reasons why their quantity of sleep is being affected.

First, let's look at the problem of falling asleep. The ability to fall asleep can be aggravated by several things. Carrying the stress you experienced during the day to bed with you is one way. Stress keeps the body tense and producing adrenaline. Adrenaline will keep you awake. Something else that inhibits sleep is the use of chemicals that stimulate your system. Those chemicals include caffeine, which is the most common and is contained in several beverages, as well as over-the-counter stimulants, and appetite suppressants. Additionally, some over-the-counter medications such as decongestants have stimulants like pseudoephedrine. Another barrier to falling asleep are abrupt noises. That's why the use of "white noise" is important in chronic fatigue. White noise is essentially any sound that is constant and masks occasional or varied sounds, such as horns, dogs barking, conversation and floors creaking, which can wake you up or prevent you from falling asleep. Another problem is light pollution. Our body needs a period of darkness to enable it to produce the brain chemical, Melatonin. Melatonin is what triggers us to fall asleep. Melatonin is only produced by the brain in response to darkness. If you leave lights on all night the body has difficulty producing melatonin and therefore we have difficulty falling asleep. I describe this inability to fall asleep in people with chronic fatigue as a state of permanent jet lag. Studies done at the Fatigue Clinic on patients who met CDC criteria for CFIDS confirmed that they were getting a high release of cortisone late in the evening—at a time when cortisone should be near or at its lowest. For people on a first shift sleep cycle, natural cortisone production is usually lowest by approximately 2 a.m. Production then starts increasing again in the early morning hours between 4 a.m. and 6 a.m. The cortisone production of people in our study, however, peaked at around 11 p.m., putting them in a state of metabolic abnormality. Since their cortisone levels were starting to go up as they were going to bed, they had trouble falling asleep and they begin to exhibit the signs of jet lag. An example of jet lag is when an American travels to Europe and tries to immediately follow a schedule based on the local time. That person experiences fatigue until their body can adjust their internal clock to change their production of cortisone. When they go to bed their bodies are producing the chemicals that help them have strength and keep awake during the day. When they get up the next morning their bodies are producing the chemicals that should be produced at nighttime, therefore they are still tired. A variation of this phenomenon appears to happen to patients with chronic fatigue syndrome. Although many patients show elevated cortisone production throughout the day because of various factors (including low blood sugar and stress), their cortisone production spikes at 11 p.m.* Sometimes my patients find it easier to fall asleep if they go to bed earlier in the evening, before their cortisone production peaks. Often patients tell me they are able to fall asleep at 9 p.m., but if they wait until 10:30 or 11:00, it's hopeless. The best treatment for this problem is a total treatment protocol for chronic fatigue syndrome that normalizes cortisone release. (Although certain medicines may help which we will discuss later).

Once asleep, there is another dilemma some patients with chronic fatigue or fatigue problems have, and that is staying asleep. Their quality of sleep is poor because they have abnormal sleep patterns or stages. Even though these patients may get seven or eight hours of sleep each night, they still awaken fatigued, and that fatigue may persist throughout the day. Also, many have frequent awakenings causing an overall decrease in the quality of sleep.

Using a concurrent EEG (electroencephalogram), doctors can monitor people who are asleep to evaluate whether they are

* Evaluation of Circadian Cortisone Release in CFIDS. E. Conley, D.O. 1992, unpublished

entering and remaining in the full cycle of each sleep stage. This method is also used to determine if someone has sleep apnea. People with sleep apnea stop breathing for a few seconds while they are asleep, usually resulting in a drop in oxygen in their bloodstream. The cause of sleep apnea is unknown, but physicians consider it to be one of the causes of constant fatigue. Patients with chronic fatigue who snore loudly or who have stopped breathing while asleep should talk to their physicians about getting a sleep study completed to determine if they have sleep apnea. (Also if you wake up at night gasping for breath). Most forms of sleep apnea are mild, though troublesome; however, in its most severe form, it can cause death. Treatment usually involves a breathing apparatus called C-PAP that keeps the person breathing and the correct percentage of oxygen in the bloodstream.

Why do people with chronic fatigue have such bad sleep quality? One of the reasons is that they seem to lack the brain neurochemicals that are needed for sleep. Our studies have shown that 56% of patients with chronic fatigue syndrome were low in Tryptophan. Tryptophan is an essential amino acid that is obtained from foods. (Tryptophan foods are: turkey, milk, soybeans, lentils and tuna). The body converts tryptophan into serotonin. Serotonin is important for helping you fall asleep and for controlling your quality of sleep. (Serotonin is also an important antidepressant neurochemical in the brain). Metabolic fluctuations may be another reason for sleep disruption. The majority of my patients with chronic fatigue have low blood sugar (hypoglycemia). Blood sugar fluctuations occur not only during the day, but also at night. While our responses to low blood sugar may not be quite as severe during the night, they still occur in response to glucose fluctuations. Low blood sugar triggers production of brain chemicals that cause the adrenal glands to release adrenaline and cortisone. This causes the liver to release stored carbohydrate in an attempt to bring the blood sugars up to normal levels. In fatigue patients, the release of adrenaline may cause stimulation of their system and disturb their sleep. The effect is the same as if someone snuck into your bedroom in the middle of the night, plugged you into an IV, and gave you caffeine without you knowing it. You would wake up a few minutes later and be unable to fall back to sleep, not knowing why.

Even while in a state of sleep, the brain is on constant vigilance, making sure the body has a normal flow of sugar and oxygen. If you wake up the same time every night, it is a telltale sign that you have low blood sugar. Often patients tell me that they wake up the same time each and every night and are unable to fall back to sleep for several hours. If this happens to you, you should suspect low blood sugar problems and try to correct them using a hypo-glycemia diet (See Chapter 11). The basis of the diet is avoidance of concentrated sweets and eating small meals or snacks frequently, this helps to stabilize the blood sugar. An idea you might try is having a very small carbohydrate snack prior to going to bed, or if you're still waking up, having one when you wake up and see if it helps you to get back to sleep. If it does, you may be hypoglycemic which is helping to disturb your sleep.

In classic depression, a patient may wake up early and be unable to fall back to sleep. I've observed a different pattern in fatigue and chronic fatigue patients. Usually patients have difficulty falling asleep and staying asleep. Once asleep, they may be able to stay asleep through the early morning, and sometimes until the early afternoon. Several other things besides the jet lag phenomenon and fluctuations in blood sugar may contribute to sleep disturbances. Factors that may affect sleep quality include lack of exercise, nutri-tional deficiencies, increased stress, high amounts of sugar in food and an imbalance of brain neurochemicals.

To improve fatigue in chronic fatigue syndrome patients, it is absolutely imperative to improve the quantity and quality of sleep. In our clinic, improving the patient's sleep quality is always one of our top priorities. What can you do to improve the quality of your sleep? First of all, make sure you get to bed early enough. It sounds peculiar, but most of us do not go to bed early enough to allow our bodies to get rested. Also, relieve the pressure on yourself about falling asleep. This, I think, is a very big pressure most of us in modern society put on ourselves. If you work, you know what time you have to get up, so you want to fall asleep as quickly as possible. The more pressure you put on yourself to fall asleep, the harder time you have doing it. Back when more people were farmers, it was not as imperative to fall asleep right away. Unless there was some task that had to be done the next day, you could sleep until you awoke rested. Or even if you couldn't sleep in, you could take catnaps throughout the day. Our schedules today don't afford us that luxury. The alarm goes off at a specific time, we work for our specific amount of time, and most of us do not nap. Many European countries have a traditional rest period during the day. A siesta is a very rational solution to lack of sleep. I think all Americans would be healthier if they had an hour or so siesta each day. Since American employers don't give their workers siestas, it's up to you to make sure you go to bed early enough so you have plenty of time to fall asleep and get eight hours of sleep. For example, if you must report for work at 5 a.m. or 6 a.m., that means you must go to bed by 9 p.m. By going to bed early you'll assure yourself of getting enough sleep, plus you may be able to beat some of the problems associated with cortisone spiking.

Another means to improve sleep is meditation. Meditation is an excellent way to slow yourself down prior to going to bed, to relieve the day's stresses from your body and mind, and to place yourself into a psychological state of relaxation, capable of drifting off to sleep. For those of you who are religious, prayer can also serve this purpose. Prayer allows you to review how your day has gone, what good you've done for other people, and your goals for tomorrow. Positive prayer lets you affirm your belief you will get better because you were meant to be healthy. In your prayer you can reaffirm that you accept your responsibility to work with people who know how to guide you back to a normal and healthful life. After a positive prayer of thanks to God for the things given to you that day and for all the truly wonderful things in your life, (including your family and material goods), you can turn your problems over to God for the night. A patient of mine recommends this prayer: "Dear God, I now place my problems into your hands. Allow me to rest, and when I awaken in the morning, I will take them back from you and do the very best I can with them." Then she takes some time to clear her mind and goes to sleep.

If you are not religious, then meditation itself is a positive way to end your day. Allow yourself to sweep the clutter from your mind and rid it of all the things you had to think about throughout the day. By easing your mind, you'll lower the tension in your body and be able to fall asleep quicker and easier. There are several meditation philosophies from which you can choose. You should experiment with various forms until you find the one that works best for you. Bedtime isn't the time to meditate on any one thing. (However, if something is troubling you, you might want to take a few minutes to meditate it). I do think it is a time to reaffirm the fact that slowly you'll become healthier, that you'll make improving your health a priority until you feel normal. More importantly, during meditation remove the day's stresses and concerns from your mind and body so you can reach a state of healing. When your mind and body become relaxed, your blood flows into all areas of your body and muscle tension decreases. Other relaxation techniques, such as self-hypnosis, are excellent means of relieving stress.

As I mentioned earlier, eating foods containing Tryptophan before going to bed may also help you fall asleep. Tryptophan is an essential amino acid that is important in the production of Serotonin, one of the brain chemicals that helps us fight depression and allows us to sleep. Since the body cannot make essential amino acids, they must be consumed. Turkey, chicken, milk and certain nuts are some foods high in tryptophan. Your grandmother was right when she said to drink a glass of warm milk before bedtime to help you sleep. (Unfortunately, many Americans are allergic to milk). (Tryptophan also is the reason why people feel tired and need to take a nap after Thanksgiving dinner). In our studies of amino acid levels in patients with chronic fatigue syndrome (CFS/CFIDS), we found tryptophan low in 56 percent. Patients with low tryptophan levels may fall asleep easier by eating foods containing tryptophan. To benefit from the drowsy reaction you get from tryptophan foods, you should eat them on an empty stomach near bedtime, or certainly in the evening. There is a study that actually measures the breakdown products of serotonin in the urine (and therefore gives us an insight into the level of serotonin in the brain). If the level is low we can use L-Tryptophan. L-Tryptophan is an amino acid available by prescription which helps with sleep disturbances by increasing the serotonin levels*. Some-times medications that have a sedative effect, such as Benadryl, help with falling asleep. The antidepressants Elevil™, Sinequan™, Pamelor™ and Desyrel™ may also aid in falling asleep, since all of those medications have sedation as a side effect. Those medica-

*Through the chemical reaction →Tryptophan →5 Hydroxytryptophan →Serotonin

tions, however, may affect quality of sleep, particularly if they are taken in high doses or if the patient is sensitive to them. Sleeping medications such as Prosom™, Ambien™, Halcion™ and Doral™, can be used to reset the time clock, but in my opinion, only patients who have intermittent sleep disturbances should use them. Those medications can be addicting and may have significant side effects, so it's best for fatigue patients with unremitting sleep disturbances to avoid them. (Ambien™ is the newest medication of this group and appears to have less addiction potential. The manufacturer recommends it be used no longer than one month. However, in studies it has been used longer without an increase in side effects and with less signs of addiction). Other antidepressants such as Prozac™, Zoloft™, Paxil™, Effexor™ and Serzone™ also may help with sleep. However, many of them may effect the quality of sleep by altering the normal stages of sleep.

Melatonin is a medication that has promise for helping chronic fatigue patients fall asleep. The melatonin currently available in health food stores is a synthetic derivative that mimics the natural product produced in the brain. The usual dosage for sleep is between 3-9 milligrams taken one hour before bedtime. Melatonin is nonaddicting, appears to be safe even in large dosages, and is used widely in Europe for treatment of jet lag and sleep disturbances. The FDA has not approved Melatonin for inducing sleep or treating sleep disturbances. (It is doubtful that the FDA will ever approve melatonin in its current form as a sleep aid. Melatonin as it currently is synthesized cannot be patented, therefore it would be pointless for any pharmaceutical company to spend the millions of dollars necessary to win FDA approval when it couldn't recoup its investment through exclusive patent rights). A review of studies done in Europe indicates that Melatonin is safe and does seem to help many patients with fatigue improve their sleep. If melatonin alone is not effective we can use it in combination with L-Tryptophan and sleep inducing herbs such as Valerian.

What if your problem is staying asleep? What can you do then? One of the first things you can do is turn on the constant sound of white noise. You can play a CD with the volume low or buy one of the machines manufactured to produce white noise. One example of white noise is the sound of gently falling rain. Some white noise machines will recreate the sound of a waterfall or the surf. You have probably noticed that when there is a steady rain tapping on your roof, it is easier to sleep. The reason you can sleep easier is because the sound is monotonous and masks other noises. When you play white noise; conversation, automobile horns and other irregular sounds are less likely to wake you up. (A cheap example of white noise is a fan). Remember though, if you think you're waking up because you stop breathing (sleep apnea), get an evaluation from a qualified sleep specialist to find out the appropriate treatment for you. We also use <u>long acting Melatonin</u> or very low doses of Sinequan™ to help patients stay asleep. Sinequan™ is a good medicine to keep you asleep, it is a very poor medicine to get you to sleep. Therefore, we often prescribe liquid Sinequan™ in combination with another medication that is shorter acting and able to help get you to sleep. The required dose of Sinequan™ varies with the patient's needs. The liquid allows us to titrate the dose to the patient's needs, this helps prevent hangover and other side effects. Most people with CFS/CFIDS require much lower doses than someone who is healthy. <u>Remember, all sleep medication and antidepressants can have side effects!</u> Consult a physician who is experienced in CFS/CFIDS before trying!

You can also enhance your sleep quality by preventing unnecessary interruptions. Make sure your children know that you need a good night's sleep and that you are not to be woken up too soon. If you need to, lock your bedroom door. If there are other interruptions that are keeping you from a quality sleep, find a way to stop them from occurring. Many times I talk with couples who have a new baby or children they worry about during the night. They would sleep more soundly if their child slept in a different room and they used a sound monitor to alert them if the child cried.

Of course, you should avoid drugs such as alcohol and caffeine, especially close to bedtime. Although alcohol has a sedative effect that allows you to go to sleep more quickly, it disrupts the quality of sleep. It is not a good medication to induce sleep. Caffeine is a stimulant that can prevent you from sleeping. Most patients with fatigue problems have difficulty breaking down caffeine in their liver. It takes smaller doses of caffeine to stimulate them than other people. Caffeine should be avoided throughout the day, particularly in the afternoon and evening.

One of the most worthwhile, if not the most worthwhile, actions you can take to get better sleep is to correct any essential vitamin, mineral and amino acid deficiencies you have. Often, after deficiencies are corrected and good sleep habits are followed, sleep problems disappear.

## AUTHOR'S UPDATE

1. L-Tryptophan: This essential amino acid is now available by prescription only. In 1989 the over the counter supplement was taken off the market by the FDA. The reason for the withdrawal was that a batch of L-Tryptophan was contaminated with amino acid E—an unnatural contaminate. This contaminate was found to be the cause of Eosinophilic Syndrome. Eosinophilic Syndrome injured many people in the U.S. and even caused death in a few. All evidence points to the fact that amino acid E caused the problem, not the L-Tryptophan. Pure L-Tryptophan appears safe when use as directed and has the potential to be very important for people with fatigue. (Not to mention the million of other people in the U.S. low in Tryptophan). It will help with sleep, by improving production of serotonin. This serotonin increase will improve depression, strengthen immunity and heighten an overall sense of well being. The lack of tryptophan is one of the reasons antidepressants are the most prescribed drugs in the U.S. (Although lack of other nutrients contribute to this "epidemic" of depression as well). There are amino acid studies available that can help evaluate if you are low in tryptophan. These should be done by a physician who is familiar with the right studies to order and how to interpret them. Otherwise they will just come back "within normal limits", and will be a waste of your time and money.

2. Light Pollution: Remember to turn the lights off in your house <u>at least</u> one hour prior to going to bed. This includes the television.

# The Bowel:
## The Most Important
## Organ of the Body

Whether you realize it or not, everything that sustains your body, with the exception of oxygen, you must take in through your bowel. The bowel is the main organ you use to relate to the environment and to the world around you. When you first hear the bowel is such an important organ you might think that is a little strange and unbelievable, especially since it is so much more apparent that you use your senses or other organs like the brain to interact with the environment. Not only is the bowel not recognized for its importance, in the United States it is seen as somewhat comical. Television and radio commercials for bowel remedies generally use humor to promote the products. People think the bowel should not be mentioned. If they do talk about it at all, they talk about embarrassing malfunctions such as gas, belching and diarrhea.

A bowel specialist I knew often told me and my fellow medical students that the bowel is the most important organ of the body. We always laughed behind her back and said, "of course she thinks the bowel is the most important organ in the body, she's a bowel specialist." However, the more that I work with patients with chronic fatigue and fatigue of all types, the more I realize that she was right. There's wisdom is those words that the bowel is the most important organ of the body. As the ancient Chinese recognized nearly five thousand years ago, "death begins in the bowel". They knew that if you did not take care of your bowel, the collapse of your body's other systems would result.

Why exactly is the bowel the most important organ in the

body? All of the other organs we consider more important, including our brain, heart, lungs, liver and kidneys need minerals, vitamins, nutrients and amino acids to function. Even the brain, which has such a dynamic functional capability in humans, must have the proper levels of oxygen, glucose, amino acids, vitamins and minerals to function. If it does not, malfunctions begin to occur. These malfunctions show up as difficulties of thought, fogginess, depression and may even become as severe as mental disease. Most people do not think of psychological illnesses as having a foundation in the physical body, but it has always been, and continues to be, my opinion that most psychological illnesses are either attributable to, or made worse by abnormalities in chemical brain function. The brain requires various chemicals, including dopamine, serotonin, nore-pinephrine, epinephrine and acetylcholine. The building blocks or raw materials for these chemicals must come in through the bowel. If we do not get that material through the bowel, then the organs that we consider to be more important than our bowel, like our brain, can't use it. Our bodies are like an island country that relies solely on one port to admit all goods. Should that port shut down for any reason, the country soon will be in deep trouble because it won't be able to receive necessary supplies. Should our port (our bowel), absorption be reduced for any reason, our body would be in deep trouble because it won't be able to receive necessary supplies (of nutrients).

Another thing most people don't realize is that the bowel is an ecosystem. In a well-regulated bowel, trillions of bacteria are necessary to keep us healthy. These bacteria are essential for the digestion of food and the absorption of vitamins, minerals and amino acids. In fact, some of the bacteria actually make vitamins such as vitamin K. Additionally, a thick layer of this so-called good bacteria helps prevent pathologic bacteria (bad bacteria) and yeast from over growing. Recent research has also found that certain bacteria produce antibiotics which actively help to kill bad bacteria. We actually produce our own natural antibiotics! Our bowel can be compared with a lawn. There are very few weeds in a thick lawn because the turf is so thick the weeds seeds can't get down in the dirt. Those seeds that do sprout get few nutrients and therefore are not able to get a foothold. Therefore there are very few weeds in a lush, thick lawn. Now, we're also finding that not only does the 'good' bacteria protect our bodies from 'bad' bacteria or pathologic invaders by acting as a barrier, but they actually fight off invaders by making antibiotics that kill or control 'bad' bacteria.

Babies are born with a sterile gut. Their bowels don't have good bacteria until their mothers seed the bacteria into them through breast-feeding. Breast milk also has nutrients that help the good bacteria to grow. Unfortunately, with the advent of formulas, more and more infants are not breast-fed. This instantly starts them off at a disadvantage since they must acquire the bacteria by other means. Infant formulas don't contain good bacteria and they contain very few of the nutrients good bacteria need to grow. Although little research has been done on the amount of good bacteria bottle-fed babies have in their bowel versus breast-fed babies, bottle-fed babies probably start off with a smaller amount and probably never catch up with their breast-fed counterparts. We know that as babies grow, good bacteria are supposed to prosper. We can help our bowels maintain the correct ecosystem by eating yogurt, which contains the good bacteria lactobacillus acidophilus. Along with yogurt we should eat other cultured foods that have nutrients that promote good bacteria growth. (Remember however to get yogurt with live bacteria. I also recommend organic yogurt so that you can avoid hormones and antibiotics that usually are in commercial cow's milk).

Good bacteria is vital for good health. It is that simple. However, our twentieth century lifestyle impedes the growth of good bacteria. We've already talked about how overgrowth of yeast and bad bacteria occurs when good bacteria is diminished (see Candida chapter). This overgrowth alters the way the bowel absorbs vitamins, minerals and amino acids. Enzyme systems need these vital nutrients to produce our energy in the Krebs cycle. After years of poor absorption of nutrients, our enzyme systems do not function as well as they should and fatigue sets in. But what does the twentieth century lifestyle have to do with diminished good bacteria counts? Why will bowel-related problems become a greater concern over the next fifty years? Antibiotics consumption is the twentieth century phenomenon that contributes the most to the problem of a sick bowel. Developed to help fight serious, life threatening infections, antibiotics have been widely used since the 1950s. Unlike the military's smart bombs, designed to hit a designated target and

67

nothing else, antibiotics hit anything that is susceptible to them—good and bad. They are like nuclear bombs that indiscriminately kill whatever is in their path. Although the antibiotic's intended target is harmful bacteria, it also hits good bacteria. Worse yet, it doesn't kill yeast and many strains of pathogenic bacteria are resistant to older antibiotics like penicillin.

Good bacteria is vital to good health. They grow in all of the body's moist areas called mucous membranes. This includes the sinuses, nose, throat, esophagus, bronchial tubes, gut, bowel, vagina and prostate. Repetitious use of antibiotics kills off much of the bowel's good bacteria. Decreased good bacteria allows yeast and bad bacteria to freely multiply. When good bacteria decrease, there is more room for bad bacteria to grow and it is easier for them to obtain nutrients. The decrease in the bowel's level of good bacteria may be compared to a lawn that has some areas of winter-kill. In the spring, the weeds will grow like wildfire in the winter-killed areas because they can get everything they need: soil, rain and sun. In the bowel, yeast and abnormal bacteria proliferate following the kill-off of good bacteria because it is the good bacteria that keeps the yeast/bad bacteria under control.

Many things happen to the body when yeast and abnormal bacteria overgrow. The most important problem is the decreased absorption of nutrients. These nutrients are vital to our health! As I discussed in earlier chapters, people are basically chemical reactions which run on enzyme systems fueled with vitamins, minerals and amino acids. These nutrient substances are essential for the proper function of the energy-generating Krebs cycle and are used as cofactors in nearly all of the body's enzyme systems. Therefore, diminished nutrient absorption results in decreased function in nearly all enzyme systems in the body. (These enzyme systems run just about everything!) So even if your diet has been excellent, (which is rare in the U.S.) you may not absorb the nutrients you need to be healthy. Remember it's not just what you eat—it's what you absorb.

People who have abnormal bowel flora (bacteria) for several years develop allergies because their bowel allows larger molecules of food to go into the bloodstream than the system is designed for. Called leaky gut, large food molecules challenge the immune system until it becomes aggravated or sensitized to certain foods, the immune system then develops antibodies, and produce symptoms of allergy. Patients who develop allergies have symptoms like stuffy nose, cough, sore throat or wheezing among others. These symptoms may cause their physicians to mistakenly think they have an infection that requires antibiotics. Another course of antibiotics however, compounds the problems these patients have since the antibiotics kill even more good bacteria. This allows further growth of yeast and bad bacteria and causes further diminishment of bowel function. The patients slowly become quite ill as this cycle of multiple antibiotics creates a downward spiral.

The lessening of the effectiveness of antibiotics may also be contributing to bowel problems. Antibiotics that were effective when they were developed some fifty years ago are now not so effective because some strains of bacteria are becoming resistant to them. (This follows the law of natural selection—survival of the fittest. The resistant bacteria that survive the antibiotics are the ones left to multiply). The "old type" of antibiotics such as erythromycin and penicillin are now being replaced by newer, stronger antibiotics, which kill more strains of bacteria and are even more deadly to good bacteria. Not only are stronger antibiotics being prescribed, they are being prescribed far too frequently. Physicians often do not think twice about prescribing an antibiotic. There are a number of reasons for that. Foremost, it is quick and easy for the physician to write a prescription rather than think about how to treat the patient's illness without antibiotics. Additionally, many patients expect to get antibiotics when they visit their doctor and may feel short-changed if they do not. An antibiotic makes them feel something is being done about their illness. Sometimes I must explain to patients why I'm not going to give them antibiotics and, sometimes, I have had patients leave the office upset because they did not receive a prescription for antibiotics. People in the United States have forgotten that you pay money to a physician to get the physicians advice; you do not pay money to the physician to get a prescription. People don't realize repetitive antibiotic use is destructive. Antibiotics are very important when they are <u>absolutely</u> needed, but very often they are not essential and actually do more harm than good. It is my opinion that the overuse of antibiotics, and the destruction they cause in the bowel and other normal floras, is and will be one of the three most serious health problems in the United States over the next generation! (The other two are stress and chemical exposure).

I read one estimate that eight hundred and fifty million courses of antibiotics were prescribed in the United States last year. That amounts to three courses of antibiotics for every man, woman and child. Since several of us did not have any antibiotics last year, that means many people took anywhere from four to ten courses of antibiotics. This statistic reminds me of a practice which I abhor. That is the practice of giving people antibiotics on a routine basis to prevent and control acne. I believe the practice ruins normal bacteria and may lead to chronic fatigue states. It's not unusual for a patient with acne to be on antibiotics for one to four years straight. A ten-day course of antibiotics for an internal infection causes enough destruction, but a six hundred day course of antibiotics for an external infection can decimate normal bacteria. Unfortunately, most patients with acne are teenagers who have very little sense of the severe health hazards their poor eating habits combined with continuous antibiotic use poses for them. My advice is, if you're on antibiotics for acne, find another way to control your acne and get off them.

Besides taking antibiotics directly, people consume antibiotics in the food they eat because of the way livestock animals are raised. Farmers routinely give antibiotics to animals in their feed to keep them healthy while they are being grown for market. The conditions under which some animals are raised stress them and make them more susceptible to disease. For instance, chickens are raised in cages in large sheds, where they never see the light of day, they don't get exercise, and more than likely their immune systems are deficient. Should a virus or bacteria invade a chicken farm, it can cause mass death. (There may be as many as ten thousand chickens in one building alone). Poultry farmers administer antibiotics to their chickens to prevent outbreaks of bacterial infections. This "preventive" measure keeps the chickens alive, also helps them to gain weight faster, which allows the farmer to take them to market quicker (therefore more profit). Very little thought is given, however, to the destruction that residual antibiotics may cause in the people who eat the chickens. Residual antibiotics show up in animal products besides chicken, including beef, pork and other commercially grown meats. Milk routinely contains some of the antibiotics farmers gave their cows to prevent udder infections.

In the United States, we are wrecking our biological systems through the indiscriminate use of antibiotics. This overuse is one of the major reasons for the fatigue problems we now face, and it will be one of the major reasons for the severe physical problems that will beset the next generation. We must stop indiscriminate antibiotic use. After reading this, some of you may become hesitant to take antibiotics when they are truly needed. <u>If you develop a severe or life-threatening infection, by all means take the antibiotic your doctor prescribes!</u> It would be foolish to die of pneumonia worrying about the level of your normal bowel bacteria. You can rebuild your normal bowel bacteria. However, when it's questionable whether you need antibiotics, you should attempt to fight off the infection using rest, supplements and good nutrition. If your doctor will not work with you on fighting an infection without antibiotics, find another doctor who will. (Most doctors do not have a clue on how to fight infections without antibiotics. Find a doctor who understands nutrition—they will be able to help.)

Besides antibiotics, two other twentieth century pharmaceutical developments—birth control pills and cortisone—contribute to destruction of the bowel's ecosystem and lead to yeast overgrowth. Birth control pills synthetically alter the normal hormonal balance in a woman. Dr. William Crook, in the widely read book *The Yeast Connection*, states that "avoidance of birth control pills is mandatory if chronic candidiasis is to be successfully controlled." He feels that the progesterone component of the pills causes changes in the vaginal mucous membrane which makes it easier for ever-present yeast to multiply and cause not only vaginitis, but associated systemic symptoms including irritability, fatigue and depression. Other mechanisms may also be involved in producing these systems, including changes in hormonal function. I have seen estimates of between seventy and one hundred million women in the United States have used birth control pills for six months or longer. They are susceptible to the symptoms Dr. Crook discusses in his book. <u>I must caution you *not* to instantly stop taking your birth control pills.</u> Pregnancy may present more short-term risks to your health than any long-term risks from birth control pills. However, you should evaluate and consider very carefully other forms of birth control especially if you have yeast problems.

Cortisone was developed in the 1940s and hailed as a breakthrough in the treatment of allergies, arthritis and inflammation. Since its development, medicine has practiced the old axiom that if a little is good, more is better. Physicians have prescribed large doses of cortisone for a number of illnesses. Unfortunately, cortisone exacerbates the bowel problems many patients have prior to taking the drug. Yeast overgrowth worsens in these patients because the yeast has receptors on it that attracts cortisone, which may actually augment yeast growth. Additionally, the large doses of cortisone usually prescribed in the United States may directly cause bowel problems. High levels of cortisone can lower immune function, thereby making it possible for abnormal bacteria, viruses and parasites to grow more freely and upset the ecosystem of the bowel. From study of the environment, you know you cannot destroy part of an ecosystem without affecting everything else in that ecosystem. You cannot cut down trees in a forest without impacting every living thing in or around that forest. Indeed, if you cut down enough of the forests, you may actually affect the entire world's climate and decrease the amount of oxygen in the air (as we now see with the destruction of the rain forest). Nor can you destroy part of your body's ecosystem without affecting how your whole body functions. When you destroy your good bacteria, yeast and bad bacteria overgrow and parasites take hold. The yeast may produce toxins which lower the immune system and make you sick directly. Yeast certainly can decrease your absorption of vitamins, minerals and amino acids. Bad bacteria can make you ill directly, causing inflammation of the bowel, diarrheal diseases, and even playing a part in arthritic diseases, such as ankylosing spondylitis and rheumatoid arthritis. Parasites can make you ill from the symptoms they cause and the part they play in allergy and immune reactions. They also contribute to arthritic type symptoms such as joint inflammation and Fibromyalgia (muscle pain).

Once you alter the normal ecosystem of your bowel, you set in motion a downward spiral that progressively pulls your health down. The spiral begins when normal bacteria are destroyed and yeast overgrows causing leaky gut that allows larger food particles into the digestive system and results in poor absorption of vitamins, minerals and amino acids. As the spiral progresses, allergies and their signs and symptoms develop. You might have a stuffy nose, congested sinuses, or bowel abnormalities such as cramping, diarrhea or constipation brought on by eating certain foods. You may even wheeze after eating some foods. A physician, believing an infection is present, may treat these symptoms by placing you on antibiotics; or you may actually develop more infections and require frequent antibiotics. The antibiotics kill more bowel bacteria, and the spiral intensifies further as amounts of abnormal bacteria and yeast increase over the years.

The immune system's job is to kill abnormal bacteria and yeast once it becomes too numerous. When your body develops anti-yeast antibodies, you may wheeze or have other symptoms whenever you eat anything with yeast or are around something that's moldy*. Plus, the yeast itself may produce antibodies that lower your immune systems. By lowering your immune system as much as possible without killing you, the yeast improves the survival rate of its next generation. Unfortunately, when your immune system decreases, viruses grow and reproduce better and you start to have viral symptoms such as recurrent sore throat, swollen glands, fatigue and cough (such as in chronic Epstein Barr infections).

Several years may pass before the poor absorption of nutrients catches up with you, but once it does, your enzyme systems and Krebs cycle won't function as well as they should. Because you aren't producing sufficient energy, you will have more fatigue and a host of other problems. Without sufficient energy, the liver doesn't detoxify the blood as it should. Metabolites start to build up, which leads to toxicity in the system. Improper amino acid absorption also means your brain doesn't have the precursors to make the brain chemicals that you need: tryptophan to make serotonin; tyrosine to make dopamine. Your brain chemicals become deficient causing difficulty with concentration and fuzzy thinking. The lack of vitamins and minerals cause your pancreas to have difficulty controlling fluctuations in your blood sugars. You may start to have abnormal sweet cravings[†] and eat more concentrated sweets, sending your blood sugar level fluctuating up and down wildly. If your pancreas is having

---

* The reason for this is that your anti-yeast antibodies cross react with other mold and yeast when you're exposed to them.
[†] Sweet cravings are usually a sign of mineral and amino acid deficiencies.

trouble controlling blood sugars, you have periods of extreme fatigue, more difficulty with lack of concentration and you reach for drugs such as caffeine, alcohol and nicotine to prop you up when you come crashing down. These drugs temporarily help you get through your workday.

At this stage of your illness, you might suffer from one or more ailments. You might develop multiple infections (such as sinus or vaginal infections) because you don't have adequate normal bacteria to protect you. These infections may require antibiotics. You might experience bowel symptoms of cramping, diarrhea and pain and get prescribed antispasmodics, which may make you drowsy or cause other symptoms. Your lungs might start to wheeze and you get a bronchodilator for your bronchial tubes, which may speed up your heart or give you other side effects. Your sinuses become congested and you have a recurrent sore throat, prompting you to take decongestants, aspirin, acetaminophen or get antibiotics for either perceived infections or real infections. Due to the abnormality in your brain chemicals, your sleep now becomes so disturbed you have difficulty sleeping though a whole night. With this disturbance in your sleep, you really start functioning poorly; no one can go too long with disturbed sleep. Sleeplessness may cause you to become moody, decrease your concentration at work, and affect your work performance to where you get reprimands, increasing your stress.

All of these changes you are undergoing produces stress that in turn produces adrenaline, one of the most toxic oxidizing agents that we know of in our bodies (Oxidation is the destruction process of nature). Constant adrenaline in your system oxidizes your enzymes, those very enzymes that are necessary for production and normal use of energy. It also builds your anxiety. Consequently, you may be diagnosed as being depressed or anxious and put on antidepressants or anti-anxiety medications. You might get skin rashes and joint pain because part of your immune system is producing massive amounts of antibodies in response to the abnormal parasites, bacteria and yeast in your system. You might even acquire an autoimmune type of disease that starts to attack your thyroid or joints, causing neck or joint pain. If your thyroid begins to malfunction, you feel even more fatigue.

Does any of this sound familiar to you? I could go on, but I hope you get the idea that once your systems begin to break down, unless you take corrective action, you start a spiral that within years, or perhaps just months, drags you down to the point where you have significant fatigue and all of the associated symptoms that go with it. (Obviously, you are not functioning so well). Now, hopefully, you see why I say the bowel is the most important organ in the body. If you had treated your bowel right, and maintained your normal bacteria levels, most of these problems would never have gotten started.

So how do we evaluate your bowel if you are sick already? Remember, it is important that you have a thorough bowel evaluation to make sure you don't have cancer. Initial evaluations involve the use of an endoscope to visually examine the interior of the bowel. In a colonoscopy, a doctor inserts an endoscope in your rectum and directs it through the bowel to view the lower gastrointestinal tract for signs of cancer or other severe abnormalities. The same procedure for the upper gastrointestinal tract is called a pandenoscopy (various names are used at different hospitals). This type of endoscopy looks down your throat, into your stomach and duodenum, to check for ulcers, inflammation and cancer. After these evaluations rule out cancer, then you should have a complete digestive stool analysis. The colonoscope and panendoscope tell little about function. They only tell structure. Many patients, if their scopes are normal are told they have "Irritable Bowel Syndrome" or "Gastritis". If you have one of these diagnoses you need a CDSA.

Available through Smoky Mountains Medical Laboratories, the complete digestive stool analysis (CDSA) assesses how your bowel is functioning by analyzing very carefully the stools you produce. The CDSA requires no work on your part other than collecting your stool samples at home. Your stools can tell a lot about your overall health, more than you ever thought possible. CDSA can tell how much good bacteria you have, if you're overgrown with yeast or bad bacteria, if you have any parasites, roughly how well you're absorbing your food, if you have too little stomach acid or too much stomach acid, if you're absorbing essential fatty acids, and if your bowel has the nutrients it needs to be healthy. Typical stool cultures don't provide a thorough enough analysis. Regular hospitals do not specialize in analyzing stool samples and therefore may not routinely look for the kinds of information needed to correctly assess bowel function. They miss meaningful information in their analyses (If you are chronically ill and feel you could benefit from a stool evaluation [I believe everyone who is ill could benefit from a complete digestive stool analysis], contact the Fatigue Clinic of Michigan for further information). After receiving results of your CDSA, we get to work on improving and restoring your normal bowel ecosystem. This restoration process may require giving you normal bacteria or medications to reduce the yeast or bad bacteria and get rid of parasites in your body. It may require giving you digestive enzymes, if you're not digesting your food well. There really is an art involved in restoring the body's ecosystem, but it is something that is vital for people with chronic illness.

One way you can protect your bowel if you've had a lot of antibiotics in the past is to begin taking normal bacteria. You must be careful which normal bacteria you take since the quality of normal bacteria varies widely. You can check with your health food store or, if you have a nutritionally oriented doctor, you can check with him or her for advice on what supplement to choose. The bacteria supplement should contain more than just lactobacillus acidophilus, because your normal ecosystem needs good bacteria other than lactobacillus. Lactobacillus bifidus, bulgaris and streptococcus faecium may also be important. The normal bacteria supplement you take should have at least three bacteria in it. You can also eat foods that have good bacteria in them to help feed your normal bacteria or reestablish the normal levels of bowel bacteria. Cultured milk products such as kefir, buttermilk and yogurt do that. You should use unsweetened yogurt, though. If you want some fruit flavor, crush up a small amount of fruit yourself and add it to the yogurt.

Perhaps the best thing you can do for your bowel and your health is to regulate your intake of antibiotics. If you are on an extended course of antibiotics, stop it unless it is for a life-threatening condition or for protection from diseases such as rheumatic fever. If you are on antibiotics for acne, discuss it with your dermatologist and find another way to control your condition. Also seek out a physician who understands nutrition, because deficiencies and lack of certain nutrients may contribute to your acne problem. When you see a physician for a respiratory ailment, make sure your physician understands that you do not want antibiotics unless they are absolutely necessary. Most health oriented physicians will work with you so you can avoid the use of antibiotics until you really require them. *As I stated before, if you have a severe or life-threatening infection, and you require antibiotics, by all means take them.* It makes little sense to die from a life-threatening infection worrying about your normal bacteria. What I'm emphasizing here is that you use antibiotics wisely. Don't be one of those patients who takes huge amounts of antibiotics when they are not needed. Remember that the bowel is the most important organ in the body and that what passes through it affects your overall health. Much can be done to restore the normal ecosystem of an ill bowel. It takes time, effort, and work, but it is well worth the effort since your bowel's good health is essential for your good health.

## IMPORTANT POINTS

1. Our bowel ecosystem is under severe attack by antibiotics, birth control pills and cortisone. These chemicals decrease the normal bowel bacteria on which the health of our bowel depends.

2. When the bowel becomes sick, it directly affects every system in our body including our immune system.

3. 90% of people seen at the Fatigue Clinic of Michigan have a sick bowel (bowel dysbiosis). If you have a significant illness of any type, more than likely you have a sick bowel as well.

4. Special stool tests can tell us the condition of your bowel. Once known it can be repaired by a physician who understands bowel ecology. However, the repair process takes time.

5. The quality of your life depends directly on the health of your bowel. If your bowel is sick it can make your life a "living hell" of pain and disease.

# ◆10◆

# **Depression**

Which comes first, the chicken or the egg? The majority of the patients with chronic fatigue immune dysfunction syndrome (CFIDS)/ chronic fatigue syndrome (CFS) who come to our clinic, have been given the diagnosis of depression by the medical establishment. Unfortunately, a large percentage of these patients were told they were only depressed and that there was nothing physically wrong. Fortunately, as knowledge about chronic fatigue syndrome improves, I am hearing less of patients being told that they are just depressed and nothing is physically wrong with them. Certainly a significant percentage of the patients that I see have depression associated with their disease, but we have to decide, which came first, the chicken or the egg? (The depression or the disease?)

A friend of mine, who is a physician in a large hospital, had the nurses come up to him rather frantically and say, "Doctor, the patient in room 157 is extremely depressed; we've got to do something. Put her on some medication as we feel depression is her problem." My friend calmly asked, "Well, what happened?" They said, "Well, she was involved in a house fire and lost her husband and lost all of her possessions and severely burned her right leg to where they're not sure it they may have to amputate." My friend looked at them rather directly and said, "If I had been in a fire and had lost my spouse and had lost my house with all my possessions and now it is possible I might lose my right leg, I would damn well be depressed."

We tend to think of depression as an illness when at times depression is a normal state of mind, such as in the incident I just described. It is normal for this lady to have been depressed. If she was not depressed, and had been sitting there smiling, that would be an abnormal psychological response.

When a person with chronic fatigue has been sick for a

78

number of years, it is a normal response that there should be some depression. The majority of patients I see are between 20 and 50 years old and should be in the prime of their lives. This is a time when they should be moving ahead in their career. They should be enjoying their personal lives, getting married, having families; or if they do have a family, being able to provide for that family in a manner that they expect, not only physically, but also psychologically. However, often the patient with chronic fatigue finds themselves in financial difficulties because of the strain the illness has placed on their resources. Not only this, but the illness has also effected the patient's ability to work. If they are still working, they're having troubles at work because of the time that they've missed. Because of the illness they are not being as productive as they once were. They certainly are not 'moving up' the corporate ladder or progressing in their career as they would like. Many of the patients have had to stop working and this has placed them in financial problems. All of these financial pressures also cause stress upon the family. Not only that, but the patients that I see feel a significant amount of stress because they worry that they are not being as good of a parent or spouse as they would like to be. They can't do the things that they used to do with their children or spouse. They feel that they're neglecting their family because they're not able to do all the things they once did. We counsel these people at length to make sure they understand that even though they can't do the quantity of activities and spend the amount of time that they used to spend, they still are able to do quality time even if it's fifteen minutes a day with their children. This quality time is very important, perhaps even more important than the quantity of time they used to spend. So, for those of you with chronic fatigue syndrome, there are ways to continue to be a very important part of your family. Add to the above factors the strain of chronic illness and it's not unexpected that depression will result. It is very common for physicians to see patients with some form of depression because of chronic illness. This is widely recognized and should not be considered an abnormal psychological state of mind. If you have a chronic illness, some depression should be considered normal. We need to treat the depression, however, when we feel that it's holding back the patient's progress or if the depression becomes severe. Certainly in chronic fatigue syndrome, the number one cause of death, the only cause of death, is suicide. This is due to depression, brought on by chronic disease. In the cases of suicidal thoughts, we must treat the depression aggressively. We should not confuse the fact that the vast majority of fatigue patients are depressed because of chronic illness, not chronically ill because they are depressed. This is a very important distinction and it is a distinction that most doctors fail to draw. Depression is not causing their illness; they do not come to see the doctor and complain of fatigue because they're depressed; depression is part of the overall spectrum of the illness. Therefore, it needs to be treated as part of the illness, just like sleep disturbances or the swollen glands and muscle pain. To treat the depression as causing the whole illness is wrong!

Along with the psychological reasons we've discussed for depression in chronic fatigue syndrome, I am convinced that the physical reasons for depression are even more important and are the same reasons that depression is so widespread in the United States. (In the near future 1 out of 3 Americans will be on anti-depressants!)

A study in our clinic has shown that in nearly 150 cases of chronic fatigue syndrome, the overwhelming majority, 85 percent were low in several essential amino acids. Many of the amino acids that they were low in are the precursors for neurotransmitters in the brain. A neurotransmitter is a chemical that transmits electrical impulses between one nerve ending and another. Most people think that the nerves in our brain are connected together, like extension cords, one end fitting into the other; but this is not the case. In between our brain nerve cells are small spaces named synapses. When a nerve ending fires it sends acetylcholine (a neurotransmitter chemical) across the synapse to the next nerve ending, or to a number of nerve endings. This stimulates the nerve endings and causes them to fire. This has happened billions of times over the last minute you've been reading this book. Without the neurotransmitter acetylcholine, you would be unable to understand what you were reading. Since neuro impulses occur many trillions times per minute, small decreases in acetylcholine will cause significant problems in communication between brain nerve cells. There are two or three precursors to the brain chemicals that appear to be low in patients with CFS/CFIDS. This deficiency may explain (on a physical basis) why so many people with chronic fatigue are depressed. One essential amino acid is tryptophan. We have demonstrated tryptophan deficiencies by amino acid analysis in 56 percent of the CFS patients evaluated in one study. Low plasma tryptophan levels have been reported in depressed patients in the *Lancet* article by Carol and Mowbray, May 9, 1970, and the levels are correlated with the degree of depression. Tryptophan is the precursor to serotonin in the body. Serotonin is an important antidepressant chemical in the brain. Much has been written and said about medications which increase the serotonin in the brain. One of these medicines is one of the most prescribed drugs in the world: Prozac™. Prozac™ reduces the ability of the body to breakdown serotonin. This causes serotonin to increase in the brain. Prozac™ and medicines like it can have serious side effects however. A major reason why so many people in the U.S. are low in serotonin is tryptophan deficiency*. If you take one of the medications which block the destruction of serotonin, this allows your serotonin levels to increase and therefore may improve your depression. Increased amounts of serotonin may also improve the immune system. Dr. Nancy Klimas at the University of Miami has shown that Prozac™ seems to improve the function of the immune system in CFIDS. Tryptophan deficiency is a significant problem in chronic fatigue syndrome. The exact reasons for this are unclear, whether the people with chronic fatigue are having trouble absorbing tryptophan, or in some way are blocking the uptake of tryptophan into the brain (many amino acids compete with each other for absorption into the brain, and if you have high levels of other amino acids, they may actively compete and reduce the movement of tryptophan into the brain).

We may not be eating enough foods that are high in tryptophan at the right times. Those foods include: turkey, low-fat milk, soybeans, nuts, bananas and tuna. (Remember to avoid any of these foods however if you've been shown to be allergic to them). Also, we may not be absorbing tryptophan (see above). In any case the majority of patients with chronic fatigue are not getting enough tryptophan. Tryptophan is in foods such as chicken, milk, turkey, tuna and soy. Tryptophan requires the proper amount of stomach acid to be absorbed well. If you are low in stomach acid or have bowel

---

* If your serotonin levels are low, you will be depressed.

dysbiosis you may absorb tryptophan poorly. If so, you will eventually become depressed.

Tryptophan cannot be supplemented legally in the United States, as it was withdrawn from the market by the FDA. The reason for this withdrawal was a problem with a contaminant in tryptophan manufactured in Japan which caused several people to be injured with eosinophilic syndrome in the U.S. The FDA has never allowed tryptophan to come back into the market even though the problem has been identified as being a contaminant and not a problem with tryptophan itself*.

Another precursor to the brain chemicals in which patients with CFS/CFIDS are low is the essential amino acid phenylalanine. Phenylalanine is the precursor to tyrosine, dopamine, and the catecholamines - epinephrine and norepinephrine. Deficiency in phenylalanine may produce low levels of the important brain chemicals dopamine and the catecholamines. Symptoms of deficiency of phenylalanine include: hypothyroidism, depression, learning and memory dysfunctions, chronic fatigue and autonomic dysfunctions. (Many of these symptoms describe very well problems that people with chronic fatigue face). It has been shown that high levels of stress tend to deplete phenylalanine levels[†]. Some of you will recognize dopamine as being the brain chemical that is low in the process of Parkinson's disease. When the area of the brain that makes dopamine is slowly destroyed, Parkinson's disease ensues causing tremor, slowness of thought and movement. No one with chronic fatigue, that I have seen, has become that severe, however, milder forms of phenylalanine deficiency and thereby dopamine deficiency cause slowness in thought and difficulty with learning and memory. These symptoms are associated with cognitive dysfunction in chronic fatigue. Cognitive dysfunction occurs in nearly 80 percent of patients seen. Tyrosine, which is made from phenylalanine, serves as a precursor to the catecholamines and thyroxine (thyroid hormone). Low tyrosine levels have been associated with hypothyroidism. (This may be one reason why I see so much subtle low

---

* L-Trytophan is now available by prescription in the United States.
[†] Wurtman and Wurtman, *Nutrition and the Brain*, Volume I -IV, New York: Raven Press (1977-83) Meta Metrix Medical Laboratory, *Clinical Relevance of Abnormal Amino Acid Values and Fasting Plasma*, Jay Alexander Bralley, Ph.D.

thyroid in chronic fatigue syndrome). Tyrosine has been used as a treatment for depression*. A study at or clinic showed eighty-five percent of CFS patients studied, were low in phenylalanine and tyrosine. These deficiencies lead to a decrease in the brain chemicals—that we need for cognitive function (thinking) and fighting depression. This includes the catecholamines which are needed for proper nerve function. (Epinephrine—the other name for epinephrine is adrenaline—which is one of the catecholamines). One reason why people may be low in the amino acid phenylalanine is the fact that so many people with chronic fatigue respond to stress so strongly and stay in a stressful state for prolonged periods of time. This may actually reduce their phenylalanine stores because of the large amount of epinephrine (adrenaline) that's needed to maintain a prolonged state of stress. Remember, adrenaline is made from phenylalanine. This, then causes a decrease in the brain chemicals that would ordinarily be made from phenylalanine and may also set up a low thyroid state which worsens the fatigue. Why? Phenylalanine is the precursor to tyrosine which is the precursor to thyroxine, which is our thyroid hormone. Let me remind all of you that, we are a whole unit.

There is no dividing the head from the body or the body from the head. If we have problems with how we're absorbing our amino acids, and our phenylalanine, tyrosine and tryptophan levels go down, then our brains will not function as well as they should! (That's one of the reasons why I stated in previous chapters, the bowel is the most important organ of the body). If our brain chemicals are not being made as well as they should we're going to be depressed. We're also going to have thought and concentration problems. We may not have the amino acids to make thyroxine which causes us to develop hypothyroidism (low thyroid). This reduces our ability to produce energy even further, and reducing our overall metabolic function. If there's one thing I wish to stress to you, it is the fact that you cannot disconnect one organ system from another—<u>everything</u> in the body is connected. If you run into problems with one organ system, sooner or later it will start to pull down other areas of the body.

That has been one of the problems with medical thought in

---

* Lancet, October 18, 1980, Gedenberg American Journal of Psychiatric 137:236:80.

this country for many years, we have tried to separate people into organ parts. We have tried to cut the brain off from the body and the body off from the brain. If a person is depressed, it is automatically thought that this is a psychological illness, therefore they need psychological medications. In my opinion, this is all garbage. You cannot have depression without having physical problems, such as amino acid, vitamin and mineral deficiencies that go along with it. You cannot have problems with the brain chemicals, without having true physiologic problems, both in the brain and outside the brain. Therefore, all treatment of "psychologic illnesses" must be directed at treating both the mind and the body. You must address the physiological (physical) problems as well as the psychological problems. Treatment of chronic fatigue cannot be based on treatment of depression. You must treat depression (if it is severe), by, when possible, finding the underlying causes of the depression and fix them. If you just treat the patient with fatigue for depression, you will fail. Therefore, if your doctor has told you that you are depressed and that there's nothing physically wrong with you, don't believe them— find another doctor. Read the rest of this book.

I have hundreds of patients who have come from all over the country and have been seen at very respected medical centers, many were told there was nothing wrong with them. When we examined them for the problems that we're discussing in this book, we have found many things wrong that we have been able to correct. They have gotten significant improvement. That has been a philosophical center point for the establishment of the Fatigue Clinic of Michigan, and a philosophy of mine; we are there to help those people with fatigue who have  been told that nothing is wrong with them. Most importantly, the majority of these problems that we identify are treatable. Many of these people have been able to resume 'normal' lives.

Let's summarize, then, my thoughts on depression in chronic fatigue.

1) The depression of chronic fatigue is both physical and psychological.

2) There are a tremendous number of people with chronic fatigue who have depression, but they are depressed because of their illness; they are not ill because they are depressed.

3) These patients need treatment for their depression, but to just treat the depression with antidepressants is to doom them to failure.

4) We must treat the depression using a holistic model; that is,

    a) Find the amino acid deficiencies and improve them.

    b) Clear up vitamin and mineral deficiencies.

    c) Start them on a good hypoglycemia diet.

Additional note: Hypoglycemia will reek havoc with brain function! Very often I see depression going hand-in-hand with hypoglycemia. From my experience at the clinic, I have found the vast majority of patients with chronic fatigue have difficulty regulating their blood sugars. Many of them have wildly swinging blood sugars. When those blood sugars start to drop the patient's brain function will be altered. (Please see the chapter on hypoglycemia). The reason for this is that our brain runs on two things: oxygen and glucose. Glucose is brought to the brain by our blood stream but is developed, of course, from our food. By glucose, most people think of the simple sugar, but glucose is actually derived from many different sources. The brain depends on a steady supply of glucose and when the glucose levels start to fluctuate, brain function will fluctuate along with it. Most people are not familiar with the problems that happen due to sugar fluctuation. Unless you happen to have a diabetic in the family who receives insulin, or you have a family member who is hypoglycemic you don't know how much trouble glucose fluctuations can cause. Most people are more familiar with the symptoms that occur with changes in oxygen levels. Several years ago, I was on vacation in Aspen, Colorado and went bicycling with a group of friends. Once we were above the 11,000 foot level, many of us started to get somewhat giddy and started to laugh out loud for no reason, or laugh at things that, were we at sea level, would not have been funny. Others in our group became irritable and cranky for no apparent reason. These were all subtle changes brought on by the lowering of oxygen at that altitude. Even though it was a very small amount lower than the oxygen in the air at sea level, it was enough to cause psychological changes. Mountain climbers and others who work at high altitudes certainly can document this. Most people will have psychological changes if they get up to certain altitudes without supplemental oxygen. The same thing can happen with blood sugar fluctuations. If you start to get fluctuations in blood sugar, it can give you many of the same changes in personality that a decrease in oxygen can. Some people will become giddy but many people will become irritable, cranky and have difficulty thinking. Many will have anxiety, heart palpitations and 'panic attacks'. All of these are signs of low blood sugar. It is very common in my clinical practice to see patients with hypoglycemia have bouts of depression. Indeed, all people that come to me with a complaint of depression are checked for hypoglycemia. It's been very well established that people with chronic fatigue have difficulties regulating their sugars (glucose). We place those patients on a hypoglycemic diet. That hypoglycemic diet involves avoidance of all concentrated sweets (please see chapter 11 on hypoglycemia). Small snacks or meals every three hours help prevent fluctuations in blood sugar. Many of my patients notice significant improvement in their fatigue as we stabilize their blood sugars. This in combination with the total therapy program as we've outlined in Chapter 16.

Adrenal fatigue: Everyone with hypoglycemia has adrenal fatigue. A person simply cannot lose control of their blood sugars without the adrenals having gotten wore down. It is very important to treat the adrenal fatigue along with prescribing the hypoglycemic diet. For a detailed discussion of the treatment of adrenal fatigue see Chapters 15 and 16.

Tryptophan: It is a crime* to sell tryptophan supplements in the United States. This is so sad because millions of people could be helped by supplementation of tryptophan. It should not be a crime to sell tryptophan in the U.S.! Millions of Americans are low in tryptophan. This deficiency causes them not to make the brain hormone serotonin in adequate amounts. This deficiency of serotonin is one of the leading causes of "endogenous depression". That is depression that doesn't have an outward cause. (Examples of an outward cause would be death of loved one, divorce or bankruptcy).

Tryptophan is available in food and those people with tryptophan deficiencies should eat foods that are high in tryptophan. My experience is that supplemental tryptophan works much better than in food alone (for those people who are deficient in tryptophan).

---

* L-Tryptophan is now available in the U.S. as a prescription drug. This may help you if you have depression or a sleep problem (insomnia). Most physicians won't know that it is available or they may still, incorrectly, think that it is harmful. To get L-Tryptophan prescribed you will have to see a health conscious physician.

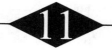

# Hypoglycemia:
# Getting Off
# The Roller Coaster

The majority of patients I see with fatigue problems have sugar problems. A small percentage of those patients have diabetes and require treatment. The vast majority of the patients, however, have what is named <u>hypoglycemia</u>. Hypoglycemia means low blood sugar. This can come about through various ways. One is through not eating for very long periods of time and eventually the body's regulatory mechanisms begin to fail and blood sugars drop low. The second is through over-excretion of insulin, either through tumors which produce insulin, or more commonly, over-reactivity of the pancreas. The third and most common mechanism is due to disregulation within the body that allows the blood sugars to fluctuate wildly. For the sake of this chapter, we're going to talk about this third problem.

How does this disregulation happen? Aren't we made to be able to eat sugar? Why, then, do we get fluctuation of blood sugar, and if our blood sugar is low, why don't we just eat more sugar, and that will keep it up, right? Wrong! The problem begins with how humans developed. We developed over thousand of years in an environment where the natural diet was very low in simple sugar. About the only simple sugar that people were able to obtain was honey, and even then that was a rarity. The everyday diet consisted of protein, complex carbohydrates (which were grains and vegetables) and fruits when available. Fruits do contain a simple sugar named fructose but also contain a large amount of fiber which slows down the release of the sugar into our system. Also, until modern times, eating fruit on a regular basis did not happen. Fruit was a luxury item, mostly during the summer. Even when fruit could be dried and eaten year-round it was still consumed in small amounts. It was just impossible to dry enough fruit to keep an entire village eating fruit on a daily basis for a long period of time. So the amount of simple sugars that humans were exposed to was small. Nature being what it is, does not build in mechanisms that are not needed. If you are not exposed to something on a regular basis, in general, you have no need to have a system handle it.

What has happened in the twentieth century is that we have exposed ourselves to a new food on an unprecedented scale. It was estimated that ancient man perhaps would eat one to two pounds of simple sugar a year. The estimates now say we eat close to 200 pounds per person per year. This is a huge increase in the amount of simple sugar that we eat versus ancient times and represents a strain on a body system that was developed to handle far less sugar.

If you eat a piece of chicken, the chicken is in a form that requires us to break it down over the course of time. We break the chicken down into units of energy and burn those units slowly. An analogy is; if you have a fire in your fireplace and you have a large log out in your backyard, you must saw a piece off the log and burn it piece by piece—that way, you're getting nice, slow energy release and therefore a nice, even, warm fire. That's really the way our bodies have been designed. We need a nice, long, even warm fire that comes from burning foods like complex carbohydrates (vegetables and grain products) and proteins. What happens when we eat some sugar, for example a candy bar? The sugar is in a form that is readily absorbable; that means that all of the sugar is absorbed into your system very quickly (usually 15-30 minutes). When this happens, our blood sugars start going up very rapidly. As our blood sugars start going up, the body senses that they are going up too rapidly and starts to produce insulin. (Insulin forces sugar into muscle cells so it can be burned as energy). We start to produce insulin like crazy because the body's trying to keep the sugar level (in our blood) within a certain range. At the time, the insulin peaks, the food is no longer still providing sugar (remember, we said all of the sugar is absorbed quickly). The candy bar is quickly absorbed but burned very quickly, and therefore, after an hour or two (dependent on the person), the blood sugars start coming back down. Only instead of coming down in a slow, orderly fashion, they start coming down very quickly (like a roller coaster). When that happens, most people get symptoms such as fuzziness of thought, irritability, fatigue, dizziness, blurred vision, and some even pass out. I'll explain how this all happens in a minute. But to go back to our fireplace analogy; it's as if you throw gasoline in the fireplace. You get a very hot, intense fire, but it's very difficult to control and it burns out relatively quickly. If you're not careful; you'll end up burning down the house instead of getting a nice, warm fire as you had intended.

How does a person with fatigue come to the point where they develop the symptoms I described of dizziness, blurred vision and irritability from hypoglycemia? This is a fairly complex course of events, which I'll try to summarize.

These symptoms don't happen the first time or even the hundredth time that you eat simple sugar. What happens over the course of years, however, is with the stress that simple sugar presents to the system, and the huge amount of sugar that we're now eating, the body must react and produce large amounts of insulin over and over again, year after year. This, in combination with the fact that we're becoming a country that is grossly deficient in minerals and vitamins. (Remember, certain minerals help control how insulin works, and also help control how we burn sugar for energy. The mineral zinc works as a cofactor that allows insulin to work. The mineral chromium is important in sugar regulation. There is considerable evidence that millions of Americans are deficient in both). Eventually, over years this repeated strain on the pancreas, in association with poor dietary habits resulting in deficiencies of vitamins, minerals and amino acids, causes the pancreas to begin to lose control over the sugars. This causes the system to over-react (although the mechanism is not totally understood). The blood sugars on certain people begin to rise and fall more quickly than they should. It has always been thought that when the blood sugars are coming down too quickly is when the symptoms ensue. (There has been some research lately that suggests that people get symptoms, not when the blood sugars were coming down, but actually when the blood sugars were rising too quickly). In either case, as those blood sugars go up and then come crashing down, people develop the symptoms that are associated with low blood sugar. These include such symptoms as fatigue, blurred vision, mental cloudiness, irritability and anxiety. Often times, when people feel these symptoms they reach for the wrong food. They have noticed (consciously or sub-consciously), that sugar seems to make them feel good when they have these symptoms. So when the sugars start crashing down, they reach for a bottle of pop, a donut or candy bar. This causes the whole process to happen all over again. The blood sugars go up wildly and an hour or two later they come crashing down causing people to reach for more simple sugar. Sometimes people reach for this simple sugar in the form of alcohol. I have yet to see, in clinical practice, an alcoholic that was not also hypoglycemic. People sometimes will also reach for drugs, such as nicotine and caffeine. That may be one reason why the coffee break was developed, to allow those people when they start getting their slump (about two to three hours after their morning meal; which was laden with caffeine and sugar) to have some more caffeine and sugar. The scenario usually goes like this: a large percentage of people in this country either skip breakfast, or when they do eat breakfast, a large percentage of their calories are simple sugar. Examples of such 'breakfasts' include; a donut and coffee, concentrated orange juice and a sugary cereal or heavily sugared muffins and mostly sugar-flavored water which we call juice drinks. Even when we do eat something that is fairly good in complex carbohydrates, such as well-made pancakes or french toast, we usually douse them with a heavy load of sugar in the form of imitation maple syrups (these are basically sugar water). In all these cases the result is the same. A couple of hours after that type of breakfast, the blood sugars come crashing down. That necessitates the person to have something else to eat (because they feel terrible). Usually, people will (if they are not knowledgeable) have some more simple sugar. This person is on a roller coaster all day. Every two to four hours they are up and then they come crashing down. They have something to eat with sugar in it; they go up, two or three hours later they come crashing down. They do this day after day, year after year. The body eventually cannot cope with this onslaught any longer, its vitamin and mineral reserves are depleted. The pancreas and adrenals are tired. The homeostasis mechanism is malfunctioning, and hypoglycemia results with the associated fatigue.

The craving for sweets in this country is overwhelming. There are those who argue that sugar is not a drug (there are even those that still argue that sugar is not harmful for you). I would agree that in <u>very small amounts</u>, in a normal person, sugar is not harmful. However, in my clinical experience, sugar acts very much like a drug. The more people eat of it, the more they appear to need and want it. Many people have psychological and physical cravings for sweets. It is very difficult to get the patient to stop eating sweets. (These three criteria define drug seeking behavior). Once we do get the patient off of this roller coaster, he/she feels considerably better, however it is usually a battle to get someone off sugar. Next to quitting smoking or alcohol, sugar is probably the hardest substance for my patients to give up. Combine that with the fact that we are sold sugar by mass marketing since the time we're able to understand. The average child watches hundreds of hours of commercials yearly. It's truly amazing how many hours a year the average child watches commercials. If you watch cartoons with your children on a Saturday morning, (other than toy commercials) you'll see the majority of foods that are advertised are sweets or junk food. This brainwashing has been going on since the 1950s and we're now in our second and third generation of it! Just try taking your children shopping and see which products they pick out. You'll be amazed, just as I am, that you can take a child shopping and they will rarely pick out a food that is healthy for them. (There are no advertisements for vegetables on Saturday morning cartoons!)

It is industry's job, when they develop a product, to try and sell us on that product. It is <u>our</u> job, if the product is junk, to avoid it (and keep it from our children)! If we do that, very soon that product will be off the market.

I do have a problem, however, with so much advertising being directed at children since children are not old enough to be able to discriminate what is good for them and what is not. I believe industry is making some steps at correcting this by paying cursory attention to making their sugar part of a "balanced breakfast" idea, however, I think it is too little—too late. The food industry really must, in the interest of public service, pay more attention to what sort of products they're putting out.

In combination with the fact that we're eating so much more sugar, we're also eating sugar at the wrong times—often by itself. Simple sugar at the end of a full meal is not as quickly absorbed and does not trigger as high of glycemic reaction (the glycemic reaction is the reaction that the pancreas must take in response to us eating the sugared food). The higher the sugar content in the food, usually the higher the glycemic reaction. However, such a large percentage of the sugar that we eat is now eaten alone. It is not uncommon for people to have coffee with sugar and a donut for breakfast. It is not uncommon for children to have some sort of heavily sweetened cereal and a sugar laden juice drink. When this happens there's very little to stop the sugar from being absorbed quickly (fiber is what slows down the absorption of sugar). In an apple there is a considerable amount of fiber in both the apple and the peel to slow the absorption of the sugar that is in the apple. In a chocolate bar there is little fiber, usually none. So we have a very unhealthy scenario; we're eating a tremendous amount of simple sugar and we're eating it at the worst possible times. Along with this, the vast majority of Americans are low in the vitamins and minerals necessary to maintain control over sugar. All of this adds up to a scenario that allows the blood sugars to go out of control and <u>millions</u> of people are affected.

Hypoglycemia has become, in my opinion, one of the major health problems in the United States. I believe this is a major contributing factor to alcoholism, juvenile delinquency, hyperactivity, depression and some learning disabilities. All of the 'diseases' I've just mentioned are severe problems in our society and the problem is getting worse. I believe that sugar problems are, along with the fatigue that ensues, one of the major drains on our productivity in the United States. There is no way of accurately measuring the amount of dollars that sugar problems cost us per year. Some estimates put this number in the trillions of dollars. That's right, <u>trillions</u>!

Another major contributing factor to hypoglycemia is adrenal fatigue (see chapter on adrenal fatigue). The adrenals are small glands above the kidneys that produce adrenaline, cortisone and many other important hormones. The adrenals become fatigued or exhausted because of the large amount of stress that we are exposed to. Also, we are deficient in the vitamins and minerals that are needed for adrenal health. When adrenals become fatigued they allow the blood sugars to fluctuate.

The treatment of hypoglycemia and adrenal fatigue go hand-in-hand. You cannot treat one without treating the other. The more hypoglycemic episodes you have, the more stress it places on the adrenals. The further wore down your adrenals become, the bigger the problem with hypoglycemia. This is another one of those episodes in the body where there develops a downward spiral. The treatment of the adrenals is outlined in the chapter on adrenal fatigue. Basically, we place the person at rest, try to have them avoid stress as much as possible and place them on the vitamins, minerals and amino acids we know are important for proper adrenal function. We start them on adrenal supplementation and control the hypo-glycemic episodes through the hypoglycemic diet. As you can proba-bly guess, the treatment of hypoglycemia is the same as the treat-ment of adrenal fatigue.

First and foremost, in treatment of hypoglycemia as it exists in chronic fatigue, we must stop the sugar roller coaster. The way to do that is: 1) Place the patient on a low simple sugar diet. 2) Make sure they eat frequently, eating every two to three hours (small amounts). Incorrectly in the past, some nutritionists have talked with patients about eating six meals a day, and although they were right, the patients become confused and think that you have to eat six actual meals a day. Most patients I've talked to will not do that because they're afraid of gaining weight. When we explain to them that they should eat their three meals a day (small) and have a snack mid-morning, mid-afternoon and early-evening, it makes more sense to them. Most patients do not gain weight, indeed, they lose weight because they're now avoiding all the high calorie—low fiber foods. For those patients who are thin and do start to lose weight, we have them increase the amount of food that they're eating. We increase the complex carbohydrates and proteins. If that does not work, we add a protein nutritional supplement drink.

In the beginning stopping all foods with simple sugars (sweets) is difficult, however, the longer you manage to stay off the sugar, the easier it becomes to avoid sweets. Also, with adults, when they start to realize how much better they feel, it becomes easier for them to avoid sweets. Sweets are pervasive in our society, so it never becomes easy. However, the benefits gained by avoiding them are usually worth it to most patients. Along with the hypoglycemic diet we treat hypoglycemia as I've outlined in the adrenal fatigue chapter. As I've stated earlier in this chapter, we also give the patient the vitamins and minerals which are known to improve adrenal function: adrenal extracts, pantothenic acid (B5), chromium (glucose tolerance factor) and zinc. (Along with a good multi-vitamin, multi-mineral and essential amino acids). If you are placed in a position where you must eat some sugar, such as someone has baked you a birthday cake, have a small piece, but make sure you do that after a full meal. We emphasize fresh vegetables in large amounts, lean proteins and complex carbohydrates. Most of all, we try to impress on the patient that they can still have fun. Eating is one of the great pleasures in life and we instruct the patients on ways of avoiding the sugar but still having fun with food. You can still have desserts using various forms of sweetener. There's considerable controversy about Aspartame at this point and I no longer recommend Aspartame to my patients because of concerns that I have about the product. So many patients have complained of headaches, blurred vision and other symptoms when they eat products with Aspartame. If you are a person that's absolutely sure you tolerate Aspartame, you can use it in small amounts (to help you stave off your sugar cravings). However, because there is a fair amount of wood alcohol in Aspartame*, I caution my patients on Aspartame. I believe there are more logical alternatives. One of those is to use a rice-base sweetener, which is a traditional Chinese sweetener; made by boiling down brown rice and using enzymes from sprouted barley to break down the starch of the rice. (First the brown rice is crushed to allow the enzymes to penetrate the hull. Next the rice is steamed and mixed with the barley enzymes and kept warm until the barley enzymes slowly digest the starch of the rice. The enzymes are then filtered out and the syrup is cooked to thicken. Usually, only brown rice and water are left as the ingredient, and there are usually no malt products remaining in the syrup, therefore, it's labeled gluten-free). I have found this to be an excellent sweetener for my patients with hypoglycemia, although, this must be used in small amounts.

* World Environmental Conference and MS 1995

Another sweetener that is used in large amounts in Japan is called "Stevia". Stevia is actually a herb that is sweet and does not break down when you cook with it (as Aspartame does). I have recently read an article that the largest percentage of diet sodas that are used in Japan are sweetened with Stevia*. Other examples of hidden sugar in foods are corn syrup, high fructose corn syrup and other sweeteners that are used to disguise the amount of sugar that is in the product.

To summarize, the treatment of the sugar roller coaster is very important in fatigue and chronic fatigue syndrome. This treatment consists of:

1) Placing the person on a hypoglycemic diet.
   a) Avoiding simple sugars.
   b) Eating small amounts more frequently.
2) Giving them the vitamins, minerals and amino acids that are necessary to allow their bodies to heal.
3) Rehabilitating the patients adrenals so that eventually they're able to stabilize the blood sugars.
4) Our complete treatment program. This point cannot be over-emphasized! Our program includes controlling sleep disturbances, improving the Krebs cycle function and improving the immune system.

## Diagnosis

The 5 hour glucose tolerance test can tell if you have hypo-glycemia. Care must be taken in the interpretation of the test. Many doctors do not know how to interpret this test properly. One major problem with the interpretation is most doctors only pay attention to how low the numbers are. They don't place enough importance on how quickly the sugars dropped and how severe the patient's symptoms were. Also, you must remember that a sugar level that may not cause problems for me, may cause them for you—or vice versa. For example: I have seen patients in my office with sugars of 27 (normal 70-110). Most people would pass out at that level. Other patients had sugars of 60 and felt horrible while many people may just feel hungry or have a headache. Also, if you drop from 120 to 60 over the course of one hour, that causes more symptoms than if you

---

* I also caution patients to avoid products that have hidden sugar, such as fruit juices which are concentrated fruit sugar without the fiber.

went from 80 to 60. <u>Everyone is an individual and you must be diagnosed and treated as an individual.</u> If you feel better after trying a hypoglycemia diet for one month—then you can be reasonably certain that you have low blood sugar regardless of what the 5 hour glucose tolerance test said.

## <u>STEVIA UPDATE</u>

1. Stevia is a herb that is 200 times as sweet as sugar, yet it doesn't have any sugar in it.
2. It is a 'cousin' to licorice, yet doesn't have a licorice taste.
3. It is not approved by the FDA in this country as a sweetener, only as a food supplement.
4. It is the most popular 'artificial' sweetener in Japan.
5. Most studies have shown it to be safe in normal use. Because it is so sweet, small amounts are needed.
6. It does not breakdown with heat. It stays sweet.
7. Relatively inexpensive.

## <u>HYPOGLYCEMIA: MAIN POINTS</u>

1. Hypoglycemia affects millions of people in the U.S. Symptoms include: fatigue, irritability and concentration difficulties. In some cases it can trigger seizures or black-out episodes. It also is a significant underlying problem in <u>alcohol and drug abuse.</u>
2. The three main causes of hypoglycemia are:
>    a. Adrenal fatigue.
>    b.The consumption of high amounts of simple sugar in this country.
>    c. Lack of essential vitamins, minerals and amino acids that the body needs to control sugar properly.
3. Hypoglycemia is a major problem in fatigue and chronic fatigue (CFS/CFIDS). A large percentage of people with fatigue have hypoglycemia. This places a terrible drain on their system. To effectively treat chronic fatigue the hypoglycemia must be treated.
4. Treatment:
>    a. Hypoglycemia diet.
>    b. Adrenal Rehabilitation: Rest, appropriate supplements and reducing stress (See chapter 15).

# Antibiotics:
# Stop The Madness

**Warning**: This chapter addresses questions about the current practices in the United States regarding antibiotics. **If you are currently on antibiotics for a serious infection, do not stop them without the advice of a physician.**

Originally when antibiotics were developed they were thought of as wonder drugs. For the first time in the history of mankind we were able to kill the bacteria that caused a wide range of diseases. These diseases included the dreaded tuberculosis and more common bacterial infections, such as strep throat. These bacterial infections had killed or injured thousands of people. Tuberculosis was known as consumption, and was the leading cause of death in the early 1900's. Strep disease caused significant death and illness by causing rheumatic and scarlet fever. Leaving into this day a generation who have scarred heart valves due to rheumatic fever. As was the case with many developments at the time, such as cortisone and nuclear energy, it was felt that these marvelous scientific breakthroughs in essence, could do no harm. Scientists, in their foolhardiness, talked about how humans would conquer all bacteria and eradicate bacterial infections from the face of the earth. They chose not to remember that bacteria had been around for over a billion years and have learned how to survive under very adverse conditions. Indeed, bacteria will be here long after human beings have gone the way of the dinosaur. Also, little thought was given to the possible side effects of antibiotics. Like children with a new toy, physicians thought that antibiotics were perfect. They thought that technology would always be able to solve all problems and if a new problem did arise, technology would simply provide the solution. Like any child with a new toy, the old therapies were soon abandoned for this new wonder drug. Soon, antibiotics were given not only for severe infections but for all infections. They were handed out like candy. They were prescribed even for infections where the physician was not sure whether it was a bacterial or a viral illness. Soon patients had grown accustomed to getting a prescription for an antibiotic, and were disappointed if they left the physician's office without an antibiotic. Few gave serious thought about the damage that was being done.

Antibiotics have saved the lives of thousands of people with serious infections. They are one of the most significant technological breakthroughs of the twentieth century. However, to ignore the fact that these same antibiotics have also caused misery and illness to thousands of people is a tragedy. We have known for years that cortisone, prescribed in too large of doses, causes severe side effects. Due to this fact, many physicians have decided not to use cortisone at all and a pendulum has swung too far in the other direction where cortisones are looked down upon by the medical community. Physicians tend to have knee-jerk reactions. Most physicians consider something as either all good or all bad, there's very few shades of grey in physician's minds. I think that's why antibiotics have been looked at as being all good, because the alternative in a physician's mind is that they are all bad: neither being the case. Antibiotics are extremely useful in life-threatening, serious infections; however, they're now being used as a convenience. As I have stated before, they are causing severe damage to thousands of people. How does the repeated use of antibiotics harm us? You must remember, there are no smart antibiotics! The military says they have smart bombs, which will miss the schools and churches and hit the target as planned. We do not have that in medicine. Antibiotics are more like nuclear bombs. When we give you an antibiotic, it kills all bacteria susceptible to it, good or bad. It does not differentiate the good bacteria from the bad. Surprisingly, most people do not understand this and when I explain this to patients they are always surprised that antibiotics kill all bacteria that are susceptible. When you are given an antibiotic, let's say for a sinus infection, it not only kills the bacteria that is causing the sinus infection, the 'bad bacteria', but it also kills good bacteria that's protecting you from infection. These good bacteria are in your bowel, vagina, prostate and anywhere you have a mucous membrane. A mucous membrane is an area that's moist, like your mouth, bowel or vagina. On the mucous membranes we have a huge number of normal bacteria. These normal bacteria serve several functions; <u>number one</u> is prevention of disease. To use an analogy, if your lawn is thick, you have very little weed problems. The reason is the weeds have no place to start; the grass gets all the moisture, sun and nutrients. However, during the wintertime if parts of your lawn are killed, then next spring the weeds will grow in those areas like wildfire. The reason is, now there's a space for them to get started. They now get the sun and nutrients and are able to thrive. Well, that's one purpose that our good bacteria serves, that is to protect our mucous membranes from bombardment by bad bacteria, parasites and viruses. With a thick lawn "of good bacteria", it's very difficult for the bad bacteria, viruses or parasites to get a foothold. The good bacteria also do a multitude of other beneficial processes. One of the most important functions takes place in the bowel. You must have good bacteria to absorb your food properly. (For a complete discussion of this, please see the chapters on bowel disorders and candida).

There has also been recent research that suggests that many of our good bacteria actually produce antibiotic-like substances that help kill bacteria or viruses*. This is an interesting new concept, which means that the good bacteria are not just passive in preventing infection, but actually are <u>active</u> in protecting you from disease. From a natural standpoint this makes a lot of sense. Since the good bacteria has a symbiotic relationship with the host, it is in the good bacteria's interest to prevent colonization by bad bacteria or viruses. Why? Because it is in the host's interest to prevent infection by invading bacteria, viruses and parasites. Synthetic antibiotics kill these good bacteria. If you have repeated courses of antibiotics or if you are on antibiotics for a long time, the antibiotic will kill enough of the good bacteria to allow yeast, viruses, and bad bacteria to get out of control. These pathogens can cause significant problems. The yeast, of course, can overgrow and block nutrient absorption in the

---

* <u>Nutritional Pearls</u> Vol 24, pp2,17, 29-33

bowel. Poor absorption of our normal nutrients over the course of several years, eventually can make us sick*. Bad bacteria can overgrow much more quickly and cause severe infections, such as infectious colitis. This is a severe form of diarrhea which occurs when certain bacteria overgrow, due to the good bacteria being killed off by antibiotics.

Another important factor that we must not forget is that it is impossible for an antibiotic to kill every one of the 'bad bacteria' in your body. If you have a lung infection and you are taking an antibiotic for it, you do not kill each and every bacteria that is causing the lung infection. You kill the majority of bacteria. However, the strongest of those bacteria survive and it is those bacteria then that are left to reproduce. Remember, in nature it's the survival of the fittest. Those "tough" bacteria are the fittest; they survive and live to reproduce the next generation.

That is the way that bacteria can develop resistance to antibiotics. Over the course of many generations, each time an antibiotic is used only the toughest bacteria survive. Those bacteria are then left for reproduction of the next generation. Since bacteria reproduce at roughly a generation an hour, you can imagine how many generations we have had over the course of the last fifty years. To use another analogy; just like in nature, natural selection is the theory that explains how animal species survive and adapt to a changing environment. If, for instance, the climate develops to where it becomes colder, it is to the animals' advantage to have thicker, longer hair. Those animals with thicker, longer hair survive better and they are the ones that are left to breed the next generation. In that generation an increased number of animals will have thicker and longer hair and they will be the ones that survive to breed the next generation, and so on. Eventually, all the animals of that species will have thick, long hair and have adapted to the changing environment.

Bacteria, even though extremely small, are animals. The same rules apply for them as any other animal in the wild kingdom. They respond and adapt to the stresses placed upon them, and we have placed tremendous stresses on them since the 1950s. These stresses are in the form of antibiotics, which have been killing vast

* Yeast also produce toxins called mycotoxins which can poison your system and cause a wide variety of symptoms. (See Candida Chapter).

numbers of weak bacteria, leaving the strong bacteria to grow and reproduce. Eventually, we create super strains of bacteria which become more and more resistant to antibiotics. As I'll explain later in this chapter, we can never stay ahead of this process. The bacteria have survived for billions of years and they will survive whatever antibiotic we can develop against them. That is why those physicians who feel that if a resistant strain of bacteria comes along all we have to do is develop another super antibiotic against it are foolhardy because we can never win. This process will reoccur and reoccur over hundreds of years until eventually there is a bacteria that we cannot develop an antibiotic against. This, of course, will have dire consequences for the human race.

One of the tragedies in the use of antibiotics is the over prescribing of antibiotics for extremely young children. Many young children have multiple allergies but the earliest allergy is usually to milk. These children develop multiple ear and throat infections and, therefore, are given antibiotics. They get these antibiotics before the normal ecosystem has been set up in their bowel and in other areas. There are a lot of children right now in this country who never developed a normal ecosystem of good bacteria in their bowel. Due to the overuse of antibiotics, at such an early age, these children have had their good bacteria decimated before they were able to develop them properly. This has caused those children to have bowel problems (leaky gut). This predisposes them to multiple allergies and will create a condition where they are sick for the rest of their life. How does this decrease in normal bacteria effect a person for the rest of their life? One way is due to the changes in bowel function. As I state in the bowel chapter, the bowel is the most important organ in the body. Everything we absorb, everything that we use in the body comes in through the bowel (except for oxygen). The bowel requires good bacteria for absorption of vital nutrients. When the good bacteria has been decimated by antibiotics, the bowel cannot absorb vitamins, minerals and amino acids (those substances which are vital for normal human function). Over the course of many years, perhaps ten or twenty years, the decrease in absorption of these vital nutrients eventually causes illness. The illness that these deficiencies cause can manifest in a number of ways. The decrease in essential nutrients (vitamins, minerals and amino acids) causes a decrease in the function of the Krebs cycle. The Krebs cycle is our energy-production mechanism (or in short, how we produce energy). This happens inside of nearly every cell in the body and all functions of the body are dependent upon the energy generated by the Krebs cycle. Enzymes are responsible for the chemical reactions that produce the energy via the Krebs cycle, and these enzymatic reactions are dependent on essential vitamins, minerals and amino acids. If you do not absorb the nutrients that you need for this energy reaction your energy production decreases and your vital functions decrease. These vital functions include your immune and endocrine function (the endocrine system is responsible for multiple regulatory processes). The endocrine system includes the thyroid, pancreas, adrenals, ovaries, testes and hypothalamus-pituitary. The destruction of our normal bacteria by antibiotics can cause far more problems than just fatigue. It sets us up for multiple recurrent infections as our immune system gets wore down from lack of vitamins, minerals and amino acids. The bacteria within our body becomes stronger, as I explained before, because the strongest bacteria have survived and are left to reproduce. There is an over-production of yeast in all areas of mucous membranes. This causes an increased production of mucous, which causes swelling of the mucous membranes, and inflammation. The congestion of these areas do not allow normal flow of mucous. Most people think of mucous as being a nuisance and only notice it if you have an overproduction. Mucous is vital, however, in protection of all of our moist membranes. Inside that mucous are large amounts of antibodies which fight off infectious organisms. The normal flow of this mucous is vital for keeping the mucous membranes healthy. A sick bowel causes a person to develop more allergies. This I discuss in other chapters in detail, but basically with the bowel having increased amounts of bad bacteria, yeast and parasites, it may become what is termed "leaky". This means that it allows absorption of larger molecules than normal into the bloodstream. The bowel is designed to absorb molecules of only certain size. Only these size molecules usually gain access to the bloodstream. When larger molecules than those are absorbed, the bloodstream does not accept them well. The body starts to recognize them as being abnormal and starts to produce antibodies against the large food molecules.

These antibodies are what causes the symptoms that we generally associate with allergies. As you build more and more antibodies to a food it triggers an antibody antigen reaction (when you eat that food). This in turn triggers histamine release causing congesting, wheezing, diarrhea and the other symptoms that can occur with food allergies. This constant congestion hinders the person in fighting off infections by obstructing the normal flow of mucous and contributes to the development of more infections. The person then gets more antibiotics causing the whole cycle to repeat itself.

The widespread overuse of antibiotics in this country is a significant contributing factor to a number of diseases which we now find running rampant through our society. Those include chronic sinusitis, vaginitis, prostatitis, asthma, irritable bowel syndrome and autoimmune diseases of all types (including lupus, rheumatoid arthritis, thyroiditis, scleroderma, sarcoidosis and other autoimmune-type reactions). It is my firm belief that unless we control how we're using antibiotics and begin to use them on a more rational basis, the next generation will be overwhelmed with autoimmune disease, allergies and fatigue. The number of patients with fatigue and chronic fatigue syndrome will continue to increase in dramatic fashion over the next generation as the scenario that I have just described plays itself out.

## <u>SUMMARY OF KEY POINTS IN THIS CHAPTER</u>

1. Antibiotics are life-saving medications when used properly.

2. Antibiotics are being over prescribed and over utilized in this country at an astounding rate (Up to 850 million doses a year).

3. The overuse of antibiotics are a significant contributing factor to the development of fatigue, chronic fatigue syndrome, autoimmune diseases, and many other chronic diseases.

4. We must work aggressively to replace the normal bacteria that has been destroyed through the use of antibiotics. We do that by supplementation of normal strains of bacteria to replace those that we have killed with antibiotics. The supplementation of good bacteria should be done routinely. (The use of foods such as yogurt is an

important part of that bowel bacteria replacement program—if you are not allergic to milk).

5. It is important that you realize that you should not quit your antibiotics if you are currently on them—without checking with a physician, nor should you refuse antibiotics from your physician if you have a <u>severe infection</u>. It makes little sense to die of pneumonia because you're concerned about your normal bacteria. However, you should avoid antibiotics whenever possible. That is to say, you should avoid them for minor infections and viral infections. Take them only if your infections are severe. After every course of antibiotics, you should work aggressively to replace the normal bacteria in your body. This means oral supplementation for your bowel and vaginal supplementation for rebuilding normal bacteria in the vagina. You should also favor those foods that help restore the normal bacterial balance in the body. These foods include yogurt and others made with live cultures.

6. If you or a loved one is on antibiotics for acne—stop them. Work with your dermatologist to find a <u>topical</u> program that works for you. The long term health consequences are not worth the short term cosmetic gain! The use of oral antibiotics for acne is not needed for over 90% of patients for whom they have been prescribed and is one of the most foolhardy health practices ever developed in the United States.

---

◆ 13 ◆

---

# Allergies:
# Why Is Allergy
# Important in Fatigue?

The vast majority of patients I see at the clinic have signifi-cant allergies contributing to their fatigue. These allergies may be inhalant, such as trees, grasses, pollens, dust-mite or mold, or these allergies may be from food. The reason we develop allergies from food is that we tend to eat the same foods over and over again. Also, these foods tend to be from the same food families. We eat the same variety of wheat year after year. It's somewhat difficult to understand but in nature there are a variety of different foods and ancient man was at the mercy of what food they could find. Therefore, it might be turkey one day and the next day some other type of wild foul, such as partridge and then another day a water foul. All of these foods appear to be the same but there's actually a subtle difference. Nowadays we eat the same foods everyday, this along with many other factors which we've created in our modern society helps to create allergy. (Another major factor is 'leaky gut'. This, we've already discussed at length in chapter 9).

Allergy can be of two types: one is acute reacting allergy named IgE. IgE is the type of allergy that most of us are familiar with. An example of that is when somebody has IgE allergy to strawber-ries. They eat strawberries and within a few minutes develop red-ness of their eyes, tightness of the chest, difficulty breathing and rash. It is pretty clear to everyone that this person is allergic to strawberries. The second type of allergy, however, is much more subtle and confusing (also controversial). This type of allergy is called slow reacting allergy (delayed hypersensitivity). Slow reacting allergies (IgG) tend to develop to foods that we eat commonly, such as wheat, corn, eggs, milk and oats. We may also develop allergies to other foods that we eat often. As an example, if a person loves almonds and eats almonds every day, they may develop an allergy over time to almonds. (If you have a leaky gut, it allows larger molecules of almonds into the bloodstream than the bloodstream was meant to handle. The body develops antibodies to these large molecules of almond. If this happens year after year an IgG allergy may result).

The reason this is important in chronic fatigue is that allergies cause a tremendous amount of damage to patients with fatigue. Allergies contribute to asthma. Asthma decreases the oxygen that the person takes in and increases the respiratory effort, meaning the patient has to expend more energy just to breathe. Asthma contributes to infections by causing a large amount of mucous, this mucous keeps airways congested and, therefore, they become more easily infected. Allergies cause problems in the entire respiratory tract, not just with the lungs. This includes the sinuses where increased congestion may lead to pain and difficulty with drainage. This may predispose one to repeated sinus infections requiring antibiotics. (Please see chapter on antibiotics).

Allergies also cause problems in the bowel. Allergies cause diarrhea, abdominal pain, gas and bloating. If severe they actually cause inflammation and may contribute to colitis. Allergies also play a part in wearing down the adrenal glands. This process becomes a vicious circle. When you have an allergic reaction your body produces histamine. Multiple allergic reactions eventually cause inflammation to develop due to all the histamine being released. This inflammation requires the body to produce more natural cortisone to try and control the inflammation. Cortisone is produced by the adrenal glands. Over years, chronic allergic reactions cause the adrenals to overwork and eventually with the increased stress that are placed on them they may start to wear down (see chapter 15). This weakening of the adrenals is due to a combination of other factors we've talked about in chapter 15, such as poor nutrition and increased amounts of stress. Once the adrenals are worn down through recurrent allergic reactions they can't produce the cortisone that is needed to control the allergic reactions. The less cortisone the adrenals produce the more out of control the allergic reactions become, and the decrease in cortisone allows you to react to more allergens. This then becomes a vicious cycle. So we have a scenario that at the early stages of chronic fatigue you develop some allergies, possibly food, possibly inhalant. The adrenals must react to help control those allergies, however, you get congestion of your sinuses and lungs, also troubles with your bowel. You receive multiple courses of antibiotics for either perceived or real infections of the sinuses and/or lungs and these antibiotics start to take a toll on the bowel. Eventually, over the course of years, the bowel may become "leaky" (if it wasn't already) where it starts allowing larger molecules of foods into the bloodstream which eventually causes the person to become allergic to more foods. The bowel also becomes overgrown with yeast and bad bacteria, and therefore, stops absorbing nutrients the way that is should. The decrease in nutrients causes a slow down in the functions of the Krebs cycle. (The Krebs cycle is our energy production mechanism). As the Krebs cycle diminishes, our total amount of energy goes down and our immune system suffers along with all the other systems of our body.

## HOW DO YOU KNOW IF YOU HAVE ALLERGIES?

Allergy symptoms are not just red eyes or a runny nose; they include lung problems,   such as shortness of breath or wheezing; bowel problems, such as diarrhea, gas , bloating or heartburn; brain problems, such as foggy thinking or dizziness; ear, nose and throat problems, such as draining sinuses, runny nose, sinus pressure, pain and recurrent infections; skin problems, such as rashes, eczema, seborrhea or psoriasis.

Many people do not realize they have allergy problems, particularly if they're allergic to foods. This is because the foods we're most allergic to are the food, we eat most often. If a person has draining sinuses on a continual basis, they rarely sit down and say, "ah-a! it's because I had wheat this morning." Well, they've had wheat every morning for the last twelve years, so they never really put two and two together and make that deduction. Occasionally, people will notice it on their own and they'll come into me and they'll say, "ya know, I've noticed that when I drink milk, I start to feel congested." However, symptoms may vary from person to person. Diagnosis requires taking a detailed history and talking with the patient. We must introduce the patient to the symptoms of food allergy and have them watch their reactions to foods closely. Then the person will start to pick out times when they have reactions. Once that happens, the person becomes aware of possible allergic problems and starts noticing other changes when they eat certain foods. Millions of Americans have allergy problems. Most have allergies that they don't know they have. Why do so many Americans have allergies? The foods we eat, tend to be the same types of food, and, we tend to eat them over and over, day in and day out. There are also other things going on that cannot be that easily explained. Millions of Americans are allergic to trees, grasses or mold. These are things we have been exposed to for millions of years. They are part of our natural environment. We evolved with trees and grasses, so why now are so many millions of people allergic to them? The answer to that has to be that there are changes going on inside of us causing us to react to things that are normal in our environment, such as pollen. Our systems are getting worn down to the point where we react to things that we should not be reacting to. We'll discuss this in more detail later in this chapter.

## WHY DO SO MANY MILLIONS OF AMERICANS HAVE FOOD ALLERGIES?

One reason is that medicine has declared war on the bowel (see chapter 9 on the bowel). The main weapon we have in our attack on the bowel is antibiotics. Antibiotics destroy normal bowel bacteria and therefore change the bowel ecosystem. Severe changes to the bowel ecosystem causes the bowel to become "leaky". Leaky means allowing larger particles of food to go into the bloodstream than the bloodstream is designed to tolerate. The body recognizes these particles as foreign. Particles of this size are not supposed to be in the bloodstream, therefore, the body develops antibodies to these large food particles. (The body develops antibodies to everything that is foreign to it). The bowel is designed to allow food particles of only a certain size into the bloodstream. These small food particles do not trigger the immune system to build antibodies against them. (At least not as readily). If the bowel is "leaky" and allowing large particles of food to be absorbed into the bloodstream, these particles trigger antibody production and eventually allergic symptoms. The more the body "sees" these particles, the more antibodies are produced. That's why we become allergic to foods we eat most often. Those are the particles that the bloodstream 'sees' most often, and the antibodies to those foods are the ones that will be developed to the greatest degree. Once enough antibodies are produced to a certain food, the person will start to have symptoms. The symptoms are caused by histamine-release when the person eats that food. Histamine usually produces the symptoms described when patients describe allergic symptomatology, such as sinus congestion, sneezing, cough, wheezing and abdominal pain. This is caused by the changes that result when histamine is released. Histamine causes tissues to swell, and this swelling causes increased congestion within the mucous membranes of the tissues. This causes the person to feel "stuffed up".

## WHAT ARE THE MOST COMMON FOOD ALLERGENS?

The most common food allergens are the foods we eat most often. This happens because these are the foods that get presented to our immune system over and over again. (Remember our discussion earlier where if the bowel is injured and is allowing particles that are to large to be absorbed, these particles are being recognized by the immune system). The most common food allergens are wheat, eggs, milk, corn and oats. In our society, these are the foods we eat every day. As we talked about before, you can also develop allergies to other foods that you eat often, for instance coffee. If you have coffee everyday, you may eventually develop some allergy to coffee. This is because we're drinking coffee several times a day, day in and day out, for years on end, and coffee particles are being presented to the immune system several times a day. Eventually, enough antibodies are produced to start to cause allergic symptoms when you drink coffee (for example: sneezing, stuffy nose or wheezing).

Allergies many times begin when we are very young. Humans were meant to drink human breast milk for at least the first six months of life. Mothers milk has good bacteria in it, which allows the bowel of the infant to be colonized with good bacteria. Her milk is also nutritionally balanced and contains vital antibodies for the needs of the baby. There is evidence that the bowel of the infant is "extra leaky", (so to speak), prior to six months of age. When foods other than mother's milk is presented to the bowel during the first few months of life, the immune system is challenged by a large amount of particles which are coming through that extra leaky bowel.

One of the reasons we may have so many food allergies in this county is that it became fashionable to feed children cow's milk or soy milk instead of mother's milk. This allows particles of the cow's milk or soy milk to be presented to the infant's immune system at the developing stage. This may be one of the reasons why so many people are allergic to cow's milk. Cow's milk is becoming implicated in causing, or contributing to immune disorders, such as diabetes, (through this allergic response). A recent study has shown that children fed cow's milk too early in life may be predisposed to diabetes. Another reason for the development of food allergies early in life is that many parents start feeding their infants cereal or other foods too early, as early as two to three months. This, again, allows an influx of large particles of those foods into the infant's bloodstream, setting them up for allergy to various foods, including wheat and oats. Remember most of the infant cereals are made from wheat, oats or corn. This may, even if they do not develop allergies now, set them up for wheat, oat or corn allergy in the future.

## WHY AREN'T FOOD ALLERGIES RECOGNIZED MORE OFTEN?

The most common food allergens are the foods that we eat most commonly, usually every day. This causes symptoms to occur daily. Therefore, people may have wheezing, chest congestion or sinus congestion (drip) on a daily basis and have had so for many years. They begin to believe they have chronic sinusitis or asthma and do not really put the connection together that they eat wheat every day and this is causing them to wheeze or have sinus drainage every day. As stated before, if you are allergic to strawberries and you eat strawberries and instantly begin to wheeze, swell, and have difficulty breathing, it's not too hard to connect this to the fact that you ate strawberries. Number one, strawberries are usually something we don't eat every day, and number two is that if it happens quickly, (an IgE allergy), it is much easier to connect. If it is a food allergy of the IgG type, it becomes very hard to distinguish what is and what is not causing problems, especially if you have multiple food allergies. Let's say you're allergic to milk, corn and wheat. Since you have one or several of these foods daily, it becomes very confusing to say what foods are causing the symptoms. You may skip wheat for a day and still have sinus drainage, that's because you are also allergic to milk and corn. You may skip milk for several days and still have sinus drainage, that's because you are allergic to wheat and corn, and so on. That's where food-allergy testing becomes important, along with elimination diets, which I will explain later.

Another reason why food allergies are not recognized more often is because doctors are not taught to recognize food allergy symptoms. Doctors are not taught a lot about allergy in medical school. Many doctors still believe that a person cannot be allergic to foods, or if they are allergic to a food, certainly those allergies cannot cause the scope of problems of which the patient is complaining. There's a tremendous amount of information available on food allergies, but most doctors are not trained to deal with foods or nutrition and, therefore, tend to think of food allergies as being "all in the patient's head". Unfortunately, most doctors are so dogmatic that when presented with symptoms that they do not understand they usually cast it off as being "all in the patient's head", rather than recognizing that something real is going on and start looking for a possible cause. The third reason why food allergies are not recognized more often is because of ignorance on the part of the general public. People do not understand the foods that they're eating may be causing their symptoms. They do not understand how allergies occur, and they don't understand how to determine if they're allergic. Many people, both doctors and patients, just feel that allergies cause sniffles and they ignore the fact that allergies cause tremendous amounts of pain and suffering in this society and are a major predisposing factor to serious illness.

## ARE WE DEVELOPING MORE ALLERGIES THAN GENERATIONS PAST?

This is difficult to say with certainty but it is my feeling that we are developing significantly more allergies than in other generations. The reason for this may be severalfold. Number one: The major reason is that our systems are being worn down by the society we've created. This includes many factors: lack of vitamins, minerals, amino acids, stress and especially the assault that is being under-taken on the bowel. (See beginning of chapter).

Number two: In general, other generations were exposed to a greater variety of foods. In our society, we tend to eat certain major food groups and concentrate on those. This has been exacerbated by "fast food". Another major problem is that farmers are raising the same types of hybrid grains all across the country. Forty years ago there were multiple types of grains, and farmers basically did not raise hybrid crops. There were many different strains of crops being produced and these small genetic variances may have been impor-tant in keeping us from developing food allergies. As I stated earlier in this chapter, a person who is allergic to chicken may not be allergic to turkey, and even though these are two similar animals they are different enough where the person allergic to chicken may be able to eat turkey, duck, partridge or pheasant. We must look at raising different foods in this country and eating a wider variety of foods.

## HOW DO WE DIAGNOSE FOOD ALLERGIES?

Diagnosis is somewhat complicated for food allergies. There are multiple ways of diagnosing allergies in general.

1. The Elimination Diet: The elimination diet is based on the principle of eliminating all but a very few hypo-allergenic foods. We keep the person on that diet for two weeks, then bring back one food group every four days, determining the response of the patient to that food group. The person writes down their response and if they developed symptoms, such as sinus drainage, congestion, sore throat, wheezing, etc., they put that food group aside and they move on to the next food group. If there wasn't any symptomatology we add that to the person's basic group of foods. There are many books which go into the elimination diet in detail. See Appendix for Elimina-tion Diet Instructions.

The elimination diet allows you to play Sherlock Holmes, in that it allows you to evaluate how you feel on certain foods. This is important because I always listen to what the patient's body is trying to tell me! Also, this test is free. It does take work but in light of the fact that allergy testing can be expensive and that insurance companies hesitate to pay for allergy testing (because they have a very poor understanding of the significance of allergy testing) it is worth the effort. The elimination diet allows anybody, rich or poor, the opportunity to determine the foods they are allergic to.

2. Laboratory testing: This allows us to determine 'suspects'. That is to say that the lab tests can give us a list of possible food allergies. We then have the patient avoid those foods for three months and then reintroduce them back into their diet (one at a time). If they do not have symptoms, we allow them to eat the foods every four days as part of a rotation diet. If symptoms return, then we have them continue to avoid the food group that causes the symptoms. There is controversy among doctors whether IgG lab testing for allergies is valid. Many doctors believe that IgG testing gives too many false positives ( a false positive means that the test is positive when the patient is not truly allergic to the food). Using the information gained from IgG/IgE testing as a basis for an elimination diet usually solves this problem. I let the patients body decide. If they feel symptoms from one of the food groups that were positive on the test—I have them avoid that food group. If they do not feel symptoms, we allow them to have that food. This is a very simple solution. Testing can be important as a short-cut for people who need help finding 'suspects' or for very complicated patients.

3. Allergy injections: There are several instances when allergy injections may benefit the patient with fatigue and CFIDS. Most of the time we recommend desensitization injections for inhalant allergies. The inhalant allergies are the ones that are most difficult to avoid particularly if the patient is very allergic to dust mites and mold. Other inhalant allergies that are easier to avoid, such as ragweed or pollen, although they are a major nuisance at certain times of the year, we do not generally recommend desensitization. For food allergies I favor the use of avoidance more than desensitization injections. I usually use food allergy desensitization only for those patients who do not have the willpower to avoid the foods they are allergic to. Desensitization is very important for children for obvious

reasons as it is very difficult to maintain a good avoidance and rotation diet with a child (although it is not impossible). There are several types of desensitization injections. There are those given by traditional allergists for which they start off on a particular dose using the same dose for most people and they increase the dose over prescribed periods of time. The problem with this type of desensitization is that it is a one-size-fits-all approach, except for some changes in dose. Usually most people receive the same doses of medication and usually use the same schedules. No effort has been made ahead of time to find out what the proper neutralizing dose is for each person. The type of allergy desensitization that I favor is called provocation/neutralization.

4. Provocation/neutralization: Provocation/neutralization is the process where a physician uses a series of extracts to determine exactly what dose of the offending agent causes the symptoms. Usually this is done by skin testing intradermally, but it can be done in other ways, such as sublingually (under the tongue). The physician starts testing at dilutions that are the most dilute and slowly increases, usually by a factor of 10 until they reach the dilution that recreates symptoms in the patient. That is called the provocation dose. That confirms that the patient is allergic to the substance injected and it also allows both the doctor and the patient to determine what the symptoms are to this particular allergy. For instance, if at a particular dose, you get a stuffy nose and wheezing, you realize that this food is the food that is causing your wheezing and stuffy nose. When testing another food, if that one causes you stomach pains, then you know it is that food, not the previous one, that is causing the stomach pain. The physician then, once the provocation dose is established, continues to test you with different doses of the same extract until a neutralizing dose is found. A neutralizing dose is the dose at which your symptoms disappear. It becomes somewhat confusing to the layperson that certain doses of the same substance can both cause symptoms and also relieve symptoms. To explain further, lets say for instance that you are allergic to corn. At a certain dose of corn, you will develop symptoms. However, at another dose we are actually able to block the symptoms that were caused by the corn. Once this neutralization dose is found, then that is the dose that is used to block

the symptoms created by the allergen. This offers several advantages. 1) It is tailored to each individual: I cannot over stress the importance of this as everyone is an individual and therefore every patient's response to allergens is different. 2) The treatment is an accurately determined neutralization dose without going through months or years of injection therapy. Often times I will have patients who have gone to traditional allergists and have been on allergy injections for years until they had discovered their blocking dose. Once that blocking dose is discovered, they start to feel improved. Provocation/neutralization testing and treatment allows you to avoid months and perhaps years of wasted time. It accurately determines the proper dose for you that allows blockage of symptoms.

Patients with chronic fatigue syndrome have to be very careful when considering allergy injections. It is important that you are receiving injections from a physician who understands what is going on with CFS/CFIDS. It is also important that you are on as accurate a dose as possible. Our rule in chronic fatigue syndrome is to avoid unneeded challenges of the immune system. This is one of the reasons why we live with allergy avoidance. We do not want to continue to challenge the immune system so that it must continue to react. If you are receiving allergy injections that are not tailor made for you, you may be continuing to challenge your immune system and this can be counterproductive. The whole science of allergy injections and desensitization is constantly changing. There are several new types of allergy testing and treatment available such as enzyme potentiated desensitization (EPD) which is currently under study. More data may be forth coming in the future on EPD, however for right now, if a person with chronic fatigue or CFS/CFIDS wishes to have desensitization therapy it is my opinion that provocation /neutralization will be most effective for them. I continue, however, to prefer avoidance therapy as much as possible. If a person is allergic to six foods, we would like them not to be on blocking solutions for all six foods. We would much rather they avoid those foods and only be on blocking solutions for those allergens to which they are extremely reactive. As an example, if a person is allergic to six foods and to mold, we would like for the patient to follow an elimination diet for their foods and eventually bring those foods back into the diet in an adequate rotation. This allows them to have neutralization only for

115

the mold, assuming they are severely mold allergic. This will improve the patient's quality of life without causing a huge amount of expense and also keeps them on the least amount of blocking medicines possible.

# IMPORTANT POINTS FROM CHAPTER 13

1. Most people with severe fatigue or chronic fatigue syndrome have significant food and/or inhalant allergies.

2. Treatment of allergies is extremely important in the overall treatment program for severe fatigue and chronic fatigue syndrome.

3. Proper diagnosis and medical treatment of those allergies usually gives significant improvement.

4. The treatment of allergies is extremely important to avoid challenges to the immune system and reduce the strain on the adrenals. This will allow the immune system to calm down and may give the adrenals a chance to heal, not to mention the fact that it will improve multiple symptoms which have been plaguing you.

5. If you are going to receive allergy injections, you need to be diagnosed properly by the provocation/neutralization method and be sure to have your proper neutralization dose determined in advance.

6. It is very important that you see physicians who understand the process of provocation/neutralization

These physicians should also understand nutritional medicine, as the treatment of allergies is only part of the entire treatment program for chronic fatigue and CFS/CFIDS.

# DHEA
## (Dehydroepiandrosterone)

### 1. WHAT IS DHEA?

DHEA is a hormone produced mainly by the adrenal glands. It is the precursor to many other hormones, that's why it's been given the name 'Mother Hormone'. It is the precursor of estrogen and testosterone in humans. DHEA production is high during adolescence and reaches maximum levels when we are in our 20's. As we age, DHEA decreases. By age 80 you produce only 10-20 percent of the DHEA you produced in your 20's (Orentreich 1984). DHEA is made from pregnenolone which is made from cholesterol.

### 2. WHY DO WE BECOME LOW IN DHEA?

During times of stress the body recognizes cortisol as the more important hormone. Production is shifted from DHEA to cortisol by the cortisol 'steal' pathway (see page 54). Just like in time of war, we have our car plants produce tanks because tanks are the priority. However, in WWII we used the car plants to build tanks for so long that eventually we started to develop a car shortage! So it is with the body. This mechanism of shifting production of DHEA to cortisol was an advantage in the world as it used to be—most of our ancestor's stresses were short or intermediate term. However most of our stresses in the 20th century are long-term stresses. (See chapter 7 on stress and chapter 15 on adrenal fatigue). With production shifted away from DHEA, slowly we develop DHEA shortage (deficiency). As this develops our immunity and energy production drops.

Stress is a major epidemic in the developed world and is causing severe problems with our DHEA levels. If this trend is not reversed we will continue to become more and more ill.

It has been accepted that we also 'naturally' produce less

DHEA as we age. There are many factors involved in this. One is that due to vitamin and mineral deficiencies our adrenals wear down over time. As they wear down, our production of DHEA drops. Another reason is that as we age we slowly damage the enzymes that are necessary to make DHEA—so our production decreases. Those people with significant bowel or digestive (malabsorption syndrome) problems also may have problems with production of DHEA. Why? Because DHEA is made from cholesterol and those people have abnormally low cholesterol. When the cholesterol is extremely low, not enough precursor is available, therefore it's more difficult to make DHEA. This problem is present in a small percentage of the population, but still I see it often enough where it shouldn't be overlooked.

The overwhelming reason for low production of DHEA in people 20-50 years old is <u>STRESS.</u> It is not uncommon for me to see patients with CFS in their 20's who are severely low in DHEA. This clinically seems to affect more men than women although the way we measure DHEA in women may be misleading

## 3. HOW DO YOU KNOW IF YOU ARE LOW IN DHEA?

The best way to determine this is by doing DHEA levels in the blood or urine. Anyone with significant fatigue should have these levels done. (In my opinion, anyone with any significant long-term health problem should have DHEA levels evaluated).

The 24 hour urine evaluation is the best way of evaluating DHEA production (and adrenal health). This way we can evaluate what your body is doing over a whole day—not just one moment in time. However, I still use the blood measurement in many of my patients because insurances seem to cover the blood studies more readily. The best evaluation is the 24 hour urine before and after a shot of ACTH (adrenal stimulating hormone). This way we can see what the adrenals are producing at rest and under 'stress' (or as a patient of mine said—"when we put the pedal to the metal.") In post-menopausal women (surgical or natural) I always do the urine study—the blood study, I feel, underestimates the normal DHEA needed for this group of women. It also makes sense to check the testosterone level—since testosterone is made from DHEA. This can be done at the same time by the 24 hour urine study (Meridian labs).

## 4. WHY IS DHEA DEFICIENCY IMPORTANT IN FATIGUE AND CHRONIC FATIGUE SYNDROME?

Most patients with severe fatigue have problems with immune function. Usually this problem is in how the immune cells move (functional activity). This is one of the serious problems in CFS/CFIDS. Most people do not have a problem with decreased number of immune cells (unlike AIDS, where the problem is not enough of certain types of immune cells). Remember that immune cells are on patrol throughout the body and must move to the site of the infection/invader. Just like in a war—if you don't have the fuel available to get the tanks and troops to the front—you have problems. So it is with the body—you must be able to get the immune cells to the site of injury or infection.

DHEA is vital in stimulating our human immune system by enhancing the production of molecules such as interleukin-2, which induce T-helper cells to proliferate and by opposing the immunosuppressive effects of glucocorticoids. DHEA can modulate the functional competence of T- and B-lymphocytes which are the cells that form the backbone of the immune system and normally serve as a major defense against infections*.

DHEA is also extremely important in energy production. It has been shown in mice to actually increase the number of mitochondria (power plants) in the cell, thereby allowing the cell to produce much more energy! (Studies have taken two groups of mice—one given DHEA, the other no DHEA given, and placed them in a pool—the group given DHEA were able to swim twice as long as the group without DHEA).

DHEA is also the precursor to testosterone (the male hormone, but this hormone also plays an important role in women's health). Testosterone is important in the function of two enzymatic steps in the Krebs cycle (remember, the Krebs cycle is how we produce energy).

---

* McCoy, James L. "Immunomodulatory Properties of DHEA as a Potential Treatment for CFIDS", The CFIDS Chronicle Physicians Forum Fall, 1993.

# Influence of Testosterone on Enzymes in the Krebs Cycle (Citric Acid Cycle)

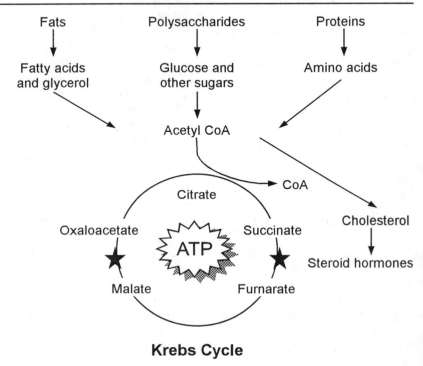

**Krebs Cycle**

Under aerobic conditions glucose enters into the Krebs Cycle via Acetyl CoA, and through a series of biochemical reactions, catalyzed in part by testosterone influenced enzymes, ATP is generated.

 Site of testosterone action on enzyme

Without adequate levels of testosterone these steps in the Krebs cycle slow down and therefore our energy production diminishes.

DHEA also improves our immunity by helping to counteract the cortisol effect. Remember, cortisol is produced in response to stress. In the short-term it improves immunity and prepares the body for inflammation that occurs with injury. (The body is getting ready to fight or run—in either case you would probably receive some injury). However with high, long-term cortisol production, (like we have these days with most of our stresses being long-term like divorce, bankruptcy, job stress, etc.) our immune system is diminished. That's one reason why most people under stress become ill (cold sores, strep throat and mono just to name a few). DHEA helps counter regulate this drop in immunity. Both by improving our immune system directly and by counterbalancing the chronic elevation in cortisol levels.

## TREATMENT OF DHEA DEFICIENCIES

In cases of fatigue and chronic fatigue syndrome, we treat DHEA deficiencies. This is done by giving the person DHEA. DHEA comes in three forms. One is injectable, which we rarely use. The two forms that we use most often are oral and topical. Both supplementation forms have their advantages and disadvantages. The oral works quickly and is easily taken. However, it also wears off quickly and since our goal of therapy is to try and maintain constant therapeutic blood levels, it is not the DHEA modality of choice at our clinic. In addition, when given DHEA orally, it has to be broken down by the liver and may be tougher on the liver than the topical cream. (To avoid this we have the patient open the DHEA capsule and sprinkle the powder under the tongue (sublingual)). I have seen DHEA capsules over the counter at health food stores, but I would caution you not to take it without a physician's guidance.

Too much DHEA can have serious side effects. Prior to taking DHEA, men should be evaluated for prostate cancer since DHEA may increase the levels of testosterone. Higher levels of testosterone when converted to dihydroxy-testosterone may cause prostate cancer to grow more quickly. Prostate examinations and PSA levels on male patients are done prior to placing them on DHEA. If you are a woman, you should be evaluated to make sure you do not have an estrogen dependent cancer prior to starting DHEA. Estrogen dependent cancers include cancer of the breast and

121

female organs. DHEA may cause an increase in estrogen levels and if you have an estrogen dependent cancer, you should not be on DHEA. You must also make certain that you do not have a lymphoma or leukemia. I do not place patients with immune cancers on DHEA. There are many reasons for you to be evaluated prior to starting DHEA and to proceed with DHEA under a physicians care. Obviously it is important that you seek council from a physician who is knowledgeable of DHEA and its use in chronic fatigue. The form of DHEA I use in my clinic is a topical cream that can be made of various strengths and is applied to the skin twice daily. This has several advantages. One is that it is absorbed slowly through the skin, allowing the skin to act as a sustained release mechanism for a slow release of DHEA into the blood stream. By applying it directly to the skin, you avoid what is called the first pass effect, that is the DHEA goes directly into the blood stream and does not have to be processed through the liver first. The disadvantages to the cream is that it is messier than pills and it more difficult to monitor with blood levels. Therefore we have to do serial urine evaluations to monitor progress of DHEA therapy.

DHEA is very important in fatigue and chronic fatigue syndrome. It is also important in many other serious illnesses. DHEA can be used with success in chronic fatigue syndrome and we use it on patients who have low levels. Again, I need to caution you, DHEA is not a magic cure, nor is it in and of itself a cure for chronic fatigue syndrome. It is another tool that we use combined with our complete treatment program.

## IMPORTANT POINTS ON CHAPTER 14-DHEA

1. Low levels of DHEA are a contributing factor to poor overall immune activity by causing a decrease in interleukin-2.

2. Low DHEA also decreases energy production by several possible mechanisms. One mechanism is a reduction in testosterone levels due to a low level of DHEA which is testosterone's precursor.

3. DHEA levels are easy to measure by blood or urine. Both DHEA and DHEA-S levels must be measured however to provide an accurate evaluation.

4. If levels are low, DHEA supplementation may be helpful. DHEA is available in pills or topical cream. At the Fatigue Clinic of Michigan the cream is the preferred therapy. Serial urine levels are done every three months to monitor for the correct dose.

5. DHEA is <u>not</u> a magical cure-all. It is helpful in fatigue <u>if</u> your levels are low and <u>if</u> you combine it with all the other therapies we have discussed. I <u>do not</u> advise using DHEA without a physicians supervision!

# Adrenal Fatigue

Perhaps no other part of our bodies are as misunderstood as the adrenals. The general public has a very poor understanding of what the adrenals do. Indeed, most people don't even know what adrenal glands are. Yet these glands are dynamos that are vital in our everyday life. Perhaps no other part of our bodies are under greater attack by modern civilization than our adrenals. The adrenals are small glands, about the size of a large hickory nut and are located right above the kidneys. Despite their small size, they are extremely dynamic. They are the source of the fight or flight response. This fight or flight phenomenon is what occurs when we are put in a position where we must either fight off an attacking animal or person, or we must be able to run away from them. The adrenals produce the hormones that are associated with fight or flight, mainly adrenaline. But the adrenals do far more. The adrenals produce the hormones that allow us to deal with stress, the most important of which is cortisol (cortisone). Most people think of cortisone as some sort of toxic drug but our bodies must produce roughly 40mg of cortisone daily or we would die. Cortisone helps us to maintain our blood pressure, enables us to fight infection, and is the main anti-inflammatory hormone of the body. For millions of years most stresses were physical. People with strong adrenals survived better (and lived to reproduce). The reason for this is that our adrenals give us, by production of adrenaline, increased strength. Adrenaline also increases our heart rate, the blood flow to our muscles (in preparation for battle), and the speed of our reflexes. Adrenaline shunts blood away from our internal organs and sends that blood to our muscles so we can have greater strength. The shunting of blood serves two purposes: 1) it gives our muscles greater strength by increasing the blood flow, 2) it reduces the amount of blood in our internal organs which decreases their chance of injury. A good way of understanding this is to think of a full water balloon. It is much easier to break a balloon that's full of water than a balloon that's only half full. An organ that's full of blood is much easier to rupture when a blow lands. Those people with good adrenal response had increased strength for fighting off another human or animal, heightened senses and increased speed for running away. The survival benefits of having strong, active adrenals in the world in which our distant ancestors lived were tremendous. It gave them a survival edge, and in nature, that's what counts. Human stresses, up until the last few hundred years, were: 1) Fighting with another human. 2) Fighting off an animal or running away from an animal. 3) Not having enough food. 4) Bad weather. All of those stresses were usually short-term, although not having enough food or bad weather could last longer, but usually never more than a few weeks. Those people with good adrenal function survived better and therefore were the ones who lived to reproduce. That's why we have adrenals today. It is important to realize though that adrenals were developed for short-term use. They are very dynamic, but they were developed for short bursts of activity. They do produce cortisone on a daily basis, but the use of the adrenals for stress was designed for short, strong bursts. Much like the boost-button on a race car. When the race driver is in a position where they can pass to gain victory, they can press the boost-button for a strong boost to their engine that increases the r.p.m.'s allowing for extra speed. However, race drivers understand that if they keep their finger on the boost-button a second too long, the increased stress on the engine will blow it. Our adrenals are like this. They were meant as a boost-button, to be used at times when we were under attack. The hormones that the adrenals produce are strong hormones and if over produced in the long-term, will cause damage to the body. Adrenaline is a very potent oxidizing agent. As we've discussed in other chapters, oxidation is the destruction process of nature. Our own adrenaline may be one of the most powerful destructive chemicals in nature. However, when you look at if from nature's point of view, it makes sense. Adrenaline was meant for short-term use, to get you away from a serious threat, so either you were able to fight off the tiger, run away from it, or you were dead. Oxidation was the least of your worries! So nature made a trade-off. It gave us chemicals that increased our strength, endurance and speed, with the trade-off being that when we use them we caused some internal destruction. Nature never intended for us to use these chemicals constantly. Cortisone is another good example. Increased production of cortisone in the short-term improves immunity, reduces inflammation and prepares us for injury during an attack by either an animal or human, in all likelihood we are going to sustain some blows that will cause injury. Cortisone reduces the inflammation caused by that injury so it doesn't get out of hand causing us to be crippled, etc., which would leave us more vulnerable to attack. Cortisone also improves immunity in the short-term, which helps us to fight off the infections that would come from wounds. However, in the long-term, high cortisone levels decrease immunity. With long-term stress and daily over production of cortisone, we actually get decreased immunity. This leaves us open to infections, including chronic bacterial and viral infections.

The stresses I have described were the stresses in the world as it used to be. That world, however, no longer exists. Our world now produces stresses that are not predominantly physical. We rarely get into physical fights with one another, and we no longer have to fight off animals. We usually have all the food we can eat, and we control our environment with furnaces and air-conditioners so that the temperature and humidity are comfortable. Our stresses now are predominately psychological. These include financial problems, job stresses, time restraints, deadlines, divorces and lawsuits, just to name a few. The body reacts the same to stress whether it is physical or psychological. Many studies have been done to show that the body also reacts to perceived stresses nearly the same as real stresses. We only have one way of reacting to stress and that is the way I've just described "fight or flight". Our adrenals respond, producing adrenaline and cortisone to get us ready to fight or to run away. So whether you're under stress from the threat of losing your job or from a tiger chasing you, your body responds nearly the same. (In fact, although you may produce more chemicals in the short-run with the tiger chasing you, over the long-run you'll produce far more chemicals from the threat of losing your job). All of our modern stresses are long-term stresses and our adrenals were designed for short-term use. This inherently produces one of the major problems that we face in the twentieth century, and that is we have created a world that is incompatible with, and hostile to our own adrenal glands. Unfortunately, it will take thousands of years for our adrenal glands to adapt to this new world. Natural selection takes time! So what happens to us in the meantime? Well, let's look at what happens to you when you put a long-term stress on your adrenals.

A) Instead of short bursts of adrenaline, you get prolonged release of adrenaline. This causes chronic elevation in your heart rate and increased muscle tension, which utilizes energy at a rapid rate. This constant muscle tension, which utilizes energy without producing work, may eventually lead to fluctuations in your blood sugar. The reason for this is that your muscles are using sugar constantly, which causes blood sugar to go down.

B) You get decreased blood flow to your organs leading to long-term mild ischemia (ischemia is the medical term which means the organ gets less blood than it needs). This may lead to spasms of the colon, bladder, or bronchial tubes, and of course, spasms cause pain and deceased function. Decreased blood flow to the liver and the kidneys will reduce how we're able to detoxify the toxins we run into on a daily basis. Decreased blood flow may be a contributing factor to irritable bowel syndrome, interstitial cystitis, asthma and many other disease processes.

C) Stress of the adrenals also increases our production of a chemical named aldosterone, which causes increased retention of sodium, water and calcium. This can cause chronic elevation in our blood pressure*. That, along with adrenaline which causes increased blood pressure by constriction of the arteries (narrowing). Together these contribute to the epidemic of high blood pressure (hypertension) in the U.S.

D) With the retention of sodium, water and calcium, we get depletion in magnesium, potassium and iodine. Magnesium is important in 375 reactions of the body, especially reactions in the Krebs cycle, the process that we use to produce energy. Decreased magnesium also causes vasospasm and bronchospasm, which contributes to hypertension and asthma. Low magnesium contributes to heart irregularities by causing spasms in the coronary arteries. Depletion of iodine can eventually lead to low thyroid.

E) Increased blood viscosity. This is due to the increased number of platelets in the blood (platelets are the blood factors that

---

* This occurs until our adrenals become exhausted, then we actually get reduced production of aldosterone causing loss of sodium (Na+) and therefore low blood pressure (hypotension), especially with standing.

help our blood to clot). This was originally useful in improving clotting. Again, if you remember, this mechanism was developed for fight or flight. That means that you're probably going to sustain some injuries, you're going to bleed and those people who clotted better, survived better. However, with psychological stresses we no longer receive injuries that cause bleeding. Now, increased platelets may contribute to stroke and heart attack by allowing our blood to clot more easily.

F) Depletion of trace minerals. This causes a reduction in SOD (super oxide dimutase), allowing for higher free radical concentrations. Decreased zinc contributes to poor insulin utilization and unhealthy prostates. Low trace minerals contribute to a tremendous amount of health problems—it would take a separate book to list all of these!

G) Elevated cortisol causes fat storage by gluconeogenesis. What this means is that when our cortisol levels are high, we are able to produce fat more effectively. This also means that if we are storing the fat, we are not burning it as energy, therefore, two problems exist. One is that we gain body fat, and the second is that we may feel fatigued because we can't burn fat as effectively for energy.

H) Chronically elevated cortisol decreases the immune system which may leave us vulnerable to recurrent bacterial or viral infections.

As you can see, the society that we have created in the twentieth century causes significant problems for our adrenal glands, which were developed in a time when we had to survive in a far different world. The response of our adrenals to the chronic stress, to which we now are exposed, is a significant contributing factor to many of the chronic diseases that ravage our country.

Above and beyond the problems caused by the chronic over-use of adrenal hormones, eventually our adrenals begin to become tired and no longer can respond appropriately to the stresses. Why do the adrenals wear down? As I described earlier, the adrenals are small glands weighing just several ounces apiece. They were meant for emergency use, they were not meant for daily over-use. Most people do not have the adrenal strength to carry them through the prolonged stresses we now face on a daily basis. It's a little bit like those small tires they give us for when we have a flat. We put the small tire on and it is good enough to get us to the service station so we can have the regular tire replaced. If you try and drive long-term on that small tire, you're not only going to destroy the tire, you're going to damage your car. This is a good example of taking something that was meant for emergency use and trying to use it on a chronic basis. As our adrenals wear down, what used to feel like mild stresses now seem severe and moderate stresses now feel overwhelming! Indeed, some people's adrenals are so worn down that just regular activities are overwhelming. This is due to the fact that they no longer have the <u>physical reserve</u> to handle stress. When this happens it isn't a <u>psychological problem</u>, it is a <u>physical problem</u>. This is one of the complaints that I have against American medicine. We try and chop people off from the head up and the head down. Anything from the head up we turn over to psychiatrists and anything from the head down we turn over to internists to have them pound with medications. In the real world there is no such thing as a strictly psychological or strictly physiological disease process. Even though most people, doctors included, think of stress as being a psychological problem, it is not. Stress is a physical problem and our response to stress and our handling of the stress relies more on the physical reserve of our adrenals then it does on our mental toughness. Indeed, our mental toughness to a large degree comes from our adrenal reserve, and if our adrenals are wore down, we cannot handle stress. The wearing down of our adrenals also results in 1) Fluctuations in mood because of uncontrolled drops in blood sugar with the associated symptoms, such as irritability, rage, fatigue and moodiness. 2) Fatigue. This is due to several mechanisms; a decrease in the Krebs cycle, a drop in cortisone production and the associated low blood sugar and mineral loss. 3) Loss of libido. Looking at this from nature's perspective, the last thing nature wants when you have a physical problem is for you to have a baby. So one of the first things that goes is our libido. The mechanical reason for this is through the Pregnenolone steal pathway (See page 54). The body steals the precursor hormone, pregnenolone, away to make cortisone, which it perceives as being the priority hormone. (Much like in the war, we converted our automobile plants to tank plants because tanks were the priority). However, if this goes on long

129

enough, pregnenolone no longer is converted into DHEA, and DHEA then is no longer made into testosterone and estrogen (at high enough levels). This has several ramifications, loss of libido, decreased energy production and loss of overall feeling of well-being. 4) Mental changes (cognitive problems) including, fuzzy thinking, depression and difficulty with short-term memory. This is due to depletion of neurochemicals and drastic fluctuations in glucose levels. Epinephrine and norepinephrine (epinephrine is our medical name for adrenaline) are brain neurochemicals that are needed for proper brain function*. 5) Increasing allergies. These include allergies to foods, pollens and our environment. These develop because of the decrease in cortisone levels as our adrenals become more and more fatigued. If you are already allergic then your reaction to allergens increase. 6) Hormone changes: It should be noted that the decrease in DHEA that comes about because of the Pregnenolone steal pathway causes a decrease in immune function and energy production. (Please see chapter on DHEA). It has been shown that DHEA is important for proper immune function and several studies have shown that DHEA is important for production of energy. Testosterone is usually considered as just a male sex hormone. The hormone that causes men to have increased body hair and sex drive. However, testosterone is much more important than that. To say that testosterone just gives men sex drive is as big an error as saying that estrogen is just important for causing a woman's menstrual cycle. Testosterone is an important catalyst for energy production. It is also important as an anabolic steroid; that means causing or directing a building up of muscle instead of a tearing down. Far too little attention has been paid to the hormone testosterone. As information becomes available we will see the supplementation of testosterone much more aggressively in men, especially post-menopausal men (andropause). It is very clear that almost all men get significant drops in their testosterone as they age. What is also becoming more clear is that what we used to expect to happen in the age range of 60-80 years, now appears to be happening in the 30-50 age group. The reason for this may very well be secondary to stress. It is now not uncommon for me to have a patient in his 30's or 40's that is low in testosterone and needing supplementation. In the first half of this

---

* Epinephrine and norepinephrine are decreased by prolonged stress.

century that would have been very unlikely.

Medicine in the past has made serious mistakes. The current dogma is that the adrenals either work or don't work. When they don't work this is called Addison's disease. (A famous example of Addison's disease is President Kennedy). This means that the adrenals are not meeting the daily requirement for the production of cortisone. However, even when the lay-person thinks about this they realize how ridiculous this dogma is. There is no other organ in the body where medicine still considers that either the organ works or doesn't work. It is ridiculous to think of the heart as either just working or not working and that there are no disease processes in-between. It is ridiculous to think of the bowel as either working or not working and there's nothing in-between. It is just as ridiculous for those physicians to cling to the outdated notion that either the adrenals work or they don't work and there are no gray areas in-between. Unfortunately, many of these physicians are Endocrinologists, which are the specialists that are meant to treat adrenal problems. (The adrenals being part of the endocrine system).

Once the adrenals are fatigued, things may proceed downhill fairly quickly. The degree to which our adrenals are drained is important. It is important to note that not all of us start off with the same adrenal strength. Adrenal function varies dependent on our stresses and nutritional status in childhood. There are also genetic factors involved, and, therefore, no two people will start off with adrenals of the same strength. Also, of course, our response to stress varies. One person may internalize stress and handle it very differently from another person whose stresses seem to run off of them like water off a duck's back. Nutritional status plays a very important part in the strength of our adrenals. Those people who had diets that were nutritionally comprised when they were young (i.e. poor eating habits) may be starting off behind the eight-ball before they even start facing the stresses of modern day life. An important factor that we also must consider is that children are facing stresses at a younger and younger age. Children are maturing much more quickly in this generation than they did in generations before. Decisions are having to be made sooner. Stresses in school begin much more quickly. Peer pressure plays an important part as does pressure obtained through television. Television inundates children with

131

the message that they should have material wealth, dress a certain way and eat certain foods. In short, we're forcing children to become adults much too quickly, and with this comes increased stress*. This all goes to point out that the degree of adrenal fatigue in one person will not be the same as in another. Dependent on the amount of stress and the strength of the adrenals to begin with, one person may develop extreme adrenal fatigue; the other person may have more mild problems. The degree of symptoms will correspond accordingly, with the person with severe adrenal fatigue having the more serious symptoms. Theses symptoms include: fatigue, decreased resistance to infections, increased allergic symptoms and auto-immune diseases (auto-immune means the body is attacking itself. Examples of auto-immune diseases are: Crohn's of the bowel, thyroiditis, rheumatoid arthritis and lupus). Ordinarily, cortisol produced by the adrenals would help control this inflammatory process, but now with the adrenals fatigued, our thyroid, joints and internal organs become damaged due to this uncontrolled inflammation. Inflammatory diseases are on the rise at alarming rates. These inflammatory diseases are not just caused by adrenal fatigue, nor are they just treated by improving the adrenals, but adrenal fatigue and the treatment of it plays an important part in the development and resolution of these "auto-immune disease processes".

So, in summary, what wears down our adrenals?

1. <u>STRESS</u>: Long-term stress and our response to it is the most important factor in wearing down our adrenals.

2. <u>LACK OF IMPORTANT VITAMINS AND MINERALS</u>: Without the proper vitamins and minerals our adrenals weaken. The lack of these essential nutrients is due to the fact that our food no longer contains them (please see discussion on the bowel). The reason for this is that our land is depleted in trace minerals and that our food is processed. This processing results in many of the vitamins and minerals being destroyed. Also, through malabsorption in our bowel

---

* A very great stress on children is the breakup of the family. Nearly 50% of parents divorce causing a tremendous amount of stress on the children at an early age. This stress lasts for years and causes untold strain of the adrenals of nearly 50% of the children in the U.S.

we are not able to absorb the vitamins and minerals that are needed for healthy adrenals. Not to mention that our dietary habits are bad. Too much junk food and not enough unprocessed foods.

3. <u>NOT ENOUGH SLEEP</u>: Rest is needed to restore the health of our adrenals. The average American gets two hours less sleep a night than they need and as discussed in the book, *The Overworked American*, we have less time available for rest and relaxation than previous generations*.

4. <u>LACK OF EXERCISE</u>: Walking reduces our response to stress, relaxes tight muscles and improves the function of the adrenals. The average American exercises far less than their parents did.

5. <u>POOR BOWEL FUNCTION (Bowel Dysbiosis)</u>: This causes decreased absorption of vital nutrients which are important to adrenal health and allows the absorption of larger molecules into the bloodstream than the bloodstream is meant to handle, leading slowly to food allergies, which further stress the adrenals.

6. <u>HYPOGLYCEMIA</u>: The increased consumption of sweets, along with decreased levels of essential vitamins and minerals eventually causes our blood sugars to swing wildly. As the blood sugars come crashing down it forces our adrenals to respond by producing adrenaline and cortisone. This release of adrenaline and cortisone causes the withdrawal of stored starch from our liver. This stored starch then helps to restore the blood sugars to normal levels. However, every time our blood sugar drops, it causes a strain on our already tired adrenals.This becomes a vicious downward spiral, as our adrenals become drained, our blood sugars fluctuate more wildly, it places greater and greater demand on our adrenals and wears them down further.

## ADRENAL RECOVERY
**IMPORTANT POINT:** <u>Adrenal rehabilitation and recovery is essential for recovery from severe fatigue and chronic fatigue syndrome.</u>

---

* Schor, Juliet B. *The Overworked American*. Basic Books, 1992. p29. According to estimates in this book. The average employed person is now in the job an additional 163 hours, or the equivalent of an extra month, a year.

The essentials are as follows:

1) <u>Rest</u>: Our adrenals recover best with rest. That's one of the reasons why treatment of sleep problems in chronic fatigue syndrome is so important. We emphasize strongly to all patients with fatigue that they get adequate rest.

2) Possibly most important is <u>stress-reduction</u>. This is difficult in our modern society, and it is too easy for the doctors just to look at the patient and say "you must reduce your stress." Rule number one is to avoid stress when possible. Sometimes we put ourselves in a stressful situation when it is not needed. I counsel my patients to evaluate their weekend times. If they have the choice between packing up the children, fighting rush hour traffic to go to an amusement park where they will have to stand in line and fight crowds of people, or finding a nice field where they can have a picnic and relax (i.e. read a book, let the children play), I counsel people to do the latter. Make changes in your life that allow you to relax!. Make sure you utilize your free time doing things that are relaxing! Do things that feel good, like a massage, reading a good book or seeing an uplifting movie. Spend quality time with your family. It does not mean you're a bad parent if you don't spend your entire weekend doting on your children! Many patients call themselves an escort service, where they're running children here, running children there. These are decisions that we make, and I recommend to you strongly to take control of your life and make those choices which will allow you to relax. Make some changes in your lifestyle.

3) <u>Simplify your life.</u> Identify those things that cause you the most stress and look at ways how you can change them. You may need to experiment to see what works for you. Our adrenals would be in great shape if we could all move to Tahiti. However, for many of us that's not practical. What is practical is that we make small changes in our lifestyle that allow us to relax. Do you really need a bigger house? Is your job truly fulfilling? Do you really need that second income or four snowmobiles and eight T.V.'s? How many new clothes or appliances do we really need? Are all these 'things' truly worth feeling the way you do? If you are 'burnt out', you really need

to take stock of what is important and decide how to change your life. One of the things that will become very important over the next decade is quality of life. Over the last twenty years we've focused on quantity of life, or as the saying goes, "They that die with the most toys, wins." The majority of people are reevaluating this philosophy. The reason is, that we are destroying ourselves in the process. If you feel absolutely lousy, have terrible interpersonal relationships and life has become a drudgery, who cares if you have a huge house or luxury automobiles? A Porsche versus a Pontiac? The next group movement in our society will be downsizing, not just on a corporate level, which is already happening, but on a personal scale. Unfortunately, everyone in the press associates this with a decreased standard of living, but it does not have to be! Our quality of life will actually improve with this downsizing as long as we don't automatically equate possessions with the quality of life.

4) <u>Handling stress better</u>: There are certain stresses in life we cannot avoid. Those stresses that we can't avoid, we need to work to handle better. I recommend meditation or prayer, or both. Meditation allows you on a daily basis to evaluate what is important in your life. It reinforces your goals and allows you to look at the 'big picture'. This can let you release many of the small things that you are stressing over right now. When you sit down and focus on what is important, you can then look at those things you're stressing over that may not be all that important and reduce your levels of stress. Prayer stresses the fact that you have help in life, that God is there and will give you help. It reinforces that everything will work out for the best. This allows you to slow down your thinking, to relax and focus in on what's important. I recommend meditation daily. If you are religious, I recommend prayer daily, especially focusing in on your favorite Bible passages. These should concentrate on relaxation, good health and strength through God. If you wish to obtain some of these prayer passages, you may want to write to the Peale Center*.

5) <u>Autoregulation</u>. This is described by my friend, Dr. Majid Ali, the author of, The Canary and Chronic Fatigue. He described it originally in his book, The Cortical Monkey and Healing. His philosophy is that

* Peale Center—Pawling, New York

when you turn off the mind, your body knows how to heal itself. Unlike many of the books you see out today stating that the mind can heal the body, he believes that the body actually has an inner sense of how it can heal itself. If you get the monkey off your back, that is, if you get the cortical thinking part of your brain to quiet down for awhile, your body can heal. For a further detailed discussion on that, I refer you to Dr. Ali's books.

6) Essential vitamins and minerals: It is clear that several vitamins and minerals are important for adrenal health. Vitamin C is a very important antioxidant and it has been known for many years that healthy adrenals are high in Vitamin C. B-Complex is also important in the function of the adrenals. Vitamin B-5 and possibly Vitamin B-15* are also important.

7) Adrenal supplements: Adrenal supplementation and/or supplementation of DHEA may be beneficial in helping your adrenals cope with illness and stress. These supplements also are important in allowing your adrenals to rebuild for the future. (Please consult the Fatigue Clinic of Michigan or your health professional for actual specific advice. Make sure you have a health professional that understands adrenal fatigue thoroughly). In ancient hunter societies, organ meats were the most prized part of the kill. Throughout ancient lore power was given to the hunter who ate a specific organ part. The hunter who ate the heart of the animal was given strength. The hunter who ate the testes of the animal gained increased sexual prowess. The adrenals were also one of the prized organ meats. The reason for this, (although the ancient people did not know exactly why) was by eating adrenals they were supplementing their own body's production of cortisone. They were also obtaining the essential vitamins and minerals necessary for adrenal health. (All of the essential nutrients were contained in the animal adrenals). Now these days we very rarely eat organ meats and unless the animal was organically grown, I would avoid these anyway. So what we do is supplement the adrenals by taking raw adrenal capsules. These are usually ground up animal adrenals processed in a beneficial way.

* DMG Dimethylgycine and is available at health food stores.

This gives us many of the nutrients necessary for adrenal strength. It also does give us a minuscule dose of cortisone and other hormones that were contained in the adrenals. Again, for a specific prescription, you need to consult an appropriate health professional. DHEA is also very important for adrenal health. (Please see the detailed discussion of DHEA in chapter 14).

8) Cortisone: If your adrenals are extremely wore down, you might benefit from cortisone in low physiologic does. This may give the adrenals some help while they are recovering. Much like a crutch when you have a broken leg, it may keep some stress off the adrenals and allow them to heal faster. This is tricky business, however, because if the dose of cortisone is too high, you will turn the adrenals off. When the adrenals are turned off, almost always, side effects are produced. If they are kept off for a long time, the adrenals begin to atrophy (decrease in size) and that is counterproductive to what we're trying to achieve. The higher the doses, the more significant the side effects and at high doses of cortisone you are virtually guaranteed side effects. Most physicians have not been trained to give cortisone in small physiologic doses and, therefore, your internist of family physician will not be familiar with this at all. They have been trained to give cortisone in large doses, or not at all. This, unless prescribed for acute allergic reactions, is the wrong way to give cortisone. (Therefore, make absolutely certain that you work with a physician who is very knowledgeable in low dose therapy).

9) Adrenal Cortical Extract: This is an injectable extract of ground-up adrenals formulized to be given either inter-muscularly or intra-venously. This is a very old type of preparation that was used mainly in the 1940s and 1950s prior to the discovery and use of oral cortisone. We started to use Adrenal Cortical Extract (ACE) at our clinic several years ago. We have had significant improvement in those patients who had mild to moderate adrenal fatigue. I like it because at low doses it is virtually free of side effects, yet gives the adrenals some help in their recovery*. (Again, it has to be used by a knowledgeable health physician).

---

* Adrenal Cortical Extract is currently unavailable in the U.S. At the time of printing, the author is unsure of when or if it will be available again.

10) <u>Avoidance of stimulants</u>: Caffeine and nicotine stimulate the adrenals. It does keep us running, however, it's like whipping a tired horse. Eventually, the horse is going to break down and then you have an even bigger problem. The continued use of caffeine and nicotine should be avoided. If you are using high doses of both, my recommendation is that you slowly decrease both. We work very hard with patients at our center to slowly get them off caffeine and nicotine (this applies to other stimulants as well). There are herbs we also use to help with caffeine withdrawal. We have seen several patients who have been addicted to cocaine, mainly because their adrenals have been worn down. They use the cocaine as a stimulant to keep them going. Treatment of adrenal fatigue should be a part of the treatment for cocaine addiction, but rarely is.

## HOW DO WE DIAGNOSE ADRENAL FATIGUE?

### 1. Adrenal Fatigue:
A) Generalized fatigue.
B) Hypoglycemia, either reactive or a low flat curve.
C) Low blood pressure with orthostatic hypotension. This means that the blood pressure drops when you stand up. Often times this is associated with getting dizzy when you bend down and get up, or when you're sitting and stand up.
D) Multiple allergies.
E) Muscle weakness in which other causes have been excluded.
F) Inability to handle physical or psychological stress.

### 2. Adrenal Testing:
Usually we do a 24-hour urine analysis before and after administration of ACTH. This will tell us how your adrenals are functioning at rest and will give us an idea what happens when they are stimulated. Or as one of my patients aptly described it, " when we put the pedal to the metal." This gives us excellent information about your adrenals over 48 hours. Along with cortisone levels we also obtain DHEA and testosterone levels. For women we also can obtain estrogen levels from this same urine sample*.

---

* We also evaluate adrenal responsiveness to exercise by drawing blood levels before and after a maximal exercise test. Your cortisol levels should roughly double. If they do not it means your adrenals are not responding appropriately to physical stress.

### 3.Blood Testing:
(This is the most common test used by Endocrinologists). Again, this is usually done before and after ACTH. The doctor evaluates the cortisone levels before, and then at one-half, and one hour after the ACTH injection. This test can be very useful if it is evaluated properly. In my experience, however, many patients who show adrenal fatigue on 24-hour urine studies have what appears to be normal pre/post ACTH stimulation by blood. They appear to be able to mount a normal stress response for a very short time, after that they decompensate quickly. Due to the fact this test misses many people with adrenal fatigue, I rarely use it.

### 4. Saliva Testing:
This is an easy way to evaluate fluctuations in cortisone levels. It has been helpful in determining if the cortisones are elevated or de-pressed at inappropriate times of day. One of our studies on chronic fatigue showed that patients with CFIDS appeared to have what best could be described as a case of permanent jet-lag. This means that their cortisones were being produced at inappropriate times for their lifestyle. Their cortisones were going up at 11:00 p.m., at a time when the cortisones should be starting to decrease. By 2:00 a.m. usually our cortisones are the lowest of the day. Their cortisones were down in the morning. This is a time when our cortisones should be the highest of the day. Their tests had the appearance of third-shifters (people working third shift, or people with jet-lag). This in spite of the fact they were following a normal 'first shift' schedule.

The best test, however, is the 24-hour urine before and after ACTH. It has consistently given us the best results and a wealth of information.

## SUMMARY

Important points to obtain from this chapter:

1. The adrenals are small glands that were originally built for emer-gency use but in the 20th century, we overuse on a daily basis.

2. Most patients with severe fatigue and chronic fatigue syndrome have adrenal fatigue.

3. The adrenals can be rehabilitated. This usually is a complex program consisting of reduction of stress, improvement of nutritional factors, meditation and/or prayer, rest and addition of natural adrenal supplements, such as desiccated adrenal capsules. Occasionally, in more severe conditions, the use of low, physiologic doses, of corti-sone are necessary until the adrenals improve.

# 16

# Treatment of Fatigue

Since the causes of fatigue are so varied and so complicated, how does one begin treating fatigue and chronic fatigue
syndrome? At the Fatigue Clinic of Michigan we take a four-prong
attack on fatigue.

## NUMBER ONE: EVALUATION OF VIRAL ILLNESS.

So many of you are told that there is no treatment for viruses.
This is wrong! There are medications available to treat viral illness,
including medications that work against Epstein-Barr, cytomegalovirus, herpes simplex virus and the human herpes virus type 6,
among others. One of the first things we do is evaluate if a person is
virally activated, and as I have explained before in the viral chapter,
that means, is there a virus that is causing significant problems for
the person right now? Activation basically means that the virus is not
dormant and is reproducing faster than the immune system can kill it.
Therefore, it's building up enough numbers to cause problems for
the person. We will never eradicate every virus from your body.
Medications are simply used to try and help control the virus while
we're working on the immune system to make it stronger. Without
the work to strengthen the immune system it would mean that you
would have to stay on the medicine forever, which is both expensive
and impractical. So, all of my patients understand that in treating viral
illness we hope to make this a short-term treatment (one year or so)
while we're working on improving the immune system. When their
immune system is strengthened we withdraw them from the
medicines we used to treat viruses. A lot of physicians still believe
that chronic fatigue syndrome is caused by a viral illness. I no longer
believe that this is the case. I believe that the viral illnesses that
accompany chronic fatigue syndrome are part of the symptom

141

complex associated with the disease, not the cause. The original problem is that the immune system is no longer working the way it should. When the immune system is not functioning the way it should, your body can no longer kill viruses as quickly as they reproduce in your body. The viral numbers build up to the point where they start to cause significant problems. It is usually at that point when the person associates that they "came down" with chronic fatigue syndrome. In reality, however, the person had been becoming sick for months or even years prior to that. The viral illness is simply the last straw that broke the camel's back. If we focus in on that last straw and neglect all the other straws that contributed to breaking the camel's back, the success of our treatment will be poor. By that I mean, if we focus in on treating a virus and treating a virus alone, then our results will be poor. We will never eradicate the virus totally from the body and once we stop medications, if nothing else has changed, you will eventually build up enough numbers of the virus to become ill again.

**What are the medications that we use to treat viral activation?**
A) <u>Kutapressin</u>™—Kutapressin™ is an extract of pig's liver developed in the 1940s. Originally, it was used in the United States for treatment of shingles, however, it was thought to be obsolete with the development of the medicine Zovirax™. It was not used in the United States since roughly the 1970s. This medicine, however, has been used in Europe for the treatment of mononucleosis, (which is caused by Epstein-Barr virus and cytomegalovirus). Some researchers from the U.S. saw that it was being used for treatment of acute mononucleosis in Europe, and brought it back to the United States in the late 1980s, and did studies to see if it would help people with Epstein-Barr in chronic fatigue. When it was found to be helpful for those patients, it became widely used at many CFIDS/CFS clinics. I've found it to be our best medicine for treatment of chronic activation of EBV, CMV and HHV-6. I've also found it to be very useful in treatment of HZV (shingles), chronic HSVI and HSVII. Since Kutapressin™ is made from pig's liver, many people mistakenly think that it contains iron, but it does not. It is a peptide (protein) with antiviral activities. It may be one way the pig fights off viruses. The pig no longer needs it, so we use it for people. The exact way

Kutapressin™ works is unknown and due to the cost that would be involved in identifying its function, probably never will be known. Its advantages are:

1) That it is extremely safe. The only listed side effect in *The Physicians Desk Reference* (PDR), is allergy to pork.

2) It is effective. It seems to have good activity against the viruses listed above.

3) It is easy to administer. It may be given at home in small injections, self-administered daily.

Its disadvantages are:

1) Cost. It is rather expensive. It's roughly $100.00 per bottle. Usually you require two bottles per month. Some patients have had their insurances cover this since it is a prescription medication, however, many insurances do not.

2) Delivery is also another disadvantage since it does not come in pill form. You must take an injection and since there's no long-acting injection, that must be done either daily or every other day.

3) Length of treatment. This medicine usually requires a three to six month regimen to determine its effectiveness and sometimes patients may be on the medication for a year or more. It should be stated that the FDA has not approved Kutapressin™ for the treatment of chronic fatigue, nor the treatment of EBV or CMV. Since no one has the millions of dollars that it takes to get approval by the FDA for Kutapressin™ in CFIDS, and the manufacturer appears unwilling to proceed along this course, I doubt seriously this medicine will ever be formally approved by the FDA for treatment of CFS*.

B. Zovirax™—This is a medication that was originally developed in the United States for treatment of shingles and herpes simplex type II (sexually transmitted herpes). It does have some effect against

---

* Kutapressin™ is approved by the FDA for use in HZV (Shingles).

EBV and CMV. It is not the preferred treatment of either CMV or EBV. However, given the cost of Kutapressin™, sometimes we must use Zovirax™. The insurances tend to cover Zovirax™ more often so we usually only use it when the patient cannot afford Kutapressin™.

C. There are a number of new antiviral medications that have recently been released, it remains to be seen how effective they will be with EBV and CMV.

## NUMBER TWO: RESOLVING THE FUNCTIONAL BLOCKS IN THE KREBS CYCLE.

This is one of the most important aspects in treatment of CFS. These functional blocks cause a decrease in the energy available to all organ systems and therefore cause an overall decrease in organ function. (Please see the further discussion of this in chapter 5 on Krebs cycle blocks). We are able to evaluate the functional blocks through a variety of studies. These studies help to tell us where the deficiencies are that have caused the functional blocks so that we can develop treatment plans designed to improve each area of blockage. The treatment of these blocks in the past has been extremely complicated. This is due to the complex nature of the Krebs cycle and the many reactions that are involved. From our work on the Krebs cycle over the past decade, we have now developed a template where we are able to determine how best to correct the blocks. This has been a quantum leap in how we treat chronic fatigue and allows us to take anyone and evaluate where their functional blocks are and how best to treat them. This has been an exciting breakthrough as it allows for individual therapy and enables us to correct one of the major underlying problems in people with chronic fatigue syndrome*.

The Krebs Cycle tests available are not perfect. It is a beginning step to discovering what your Krebs cycle is doing and how to fix the functional blocks.

## NUMBER THREE:
## RESTORING THE ECOSYSTEM OF THE BOWEL.

As I explained in the bowel chapter, the vast majority of people with fatigue and CFIDS/CFS have severely altered bowel

---

* This is also important for all people with fatigue and those diagnosed with fibromyalgia.

ecosystems. If you are to return to long-term health and to stay healthy for the rest of your life, you must restore the normal ecosystem of the bowel. The way we accomplish this is as follows:

A) We increase the normal bacteria of the bowel. This is usually accomplished through taking supplements that include the bacteria important for normal bowel function. These include lactobacillus acidophilus and bifidobacteria, and may also include fructo-oligosaccharides (FOS). FOS is a sugar (usually derived from Jerusalem artichokes) that the good bacteria in the bowel can utilize but abnormal bacteria cannot. Restoring normal bacteria is the most important long-term treatment for healing the bowel ecosystem. Along with supplements of normal bacteria, we also encourage foods that allow for normal bacteria development. That includes foods that are high in fiber, also foods that contain good bacteria. One very good example of this is yogurt. (You must be careful what yogurt you purchase, however, as the good bacteria may be dead). Often we recommend patients make their own yogurt at home, but if this is impossible you should consider purchasing organic yogurt from a health store. Organic yogurt will not contain the antibiotics present in regular milk—this is an added benefit of organic yogurt.

B) Reduce the yeast, parasites and abnormal bacteria in the bowel. How do we accomplish this? First, we determine through a special in depth stool study, the flora of the bowel as it now exists. If you are overgrown with yeast, then we prescribe appropriate anti-yeast medicines, such as Nystatin, Diflucan™ or Sporanox™. At the same time, we evaluate for parasitic overgrowth and if parasites are present we treat those. We've also recently started to do rectal swabs to more intensely evaluate for parasitic infection. Treating abnormal bacteria is somewhat more controversial as we are unsure just what problems abnormal bacteria can cause in the bowel. I have, over the last few years, taken a much more aggressive approach in treating abnormal bacteria. My preferred route is to try to treat it naturally with herbal combinations. This accomplishes two goals. One is, it does not harm the remaining normal bacteria, and two is, it reduces the abnormal bacteria hopefully without increasing resistance. Usually these bacteria are fairly resistant to antibiotics and my experience in treating them with large doses of strong antibiotics has been poor. However, my response to treatment with herbal preparations has been good.

## NUMBER FOUR:
## WE WORK HARD TO RESTORE THE DIMINISHED FUNCTIONS OF OTHER ORGAN SYSTEMS THAT ARE WORN DOWN IN FATIGUE AND CHRONIC FATIGUE.

1.The Adrenals - The endocrine system suffers the most in patients with chronic fatigue. In that system perhaps no other organ is worn down as much as the adrenals. (Please see the chapter on Adrenal Fatigue). Treatment of adrenal fatigue is complicated but requires B-Complex, along with B-5 and Vitamin C. We add doses of a natural adrenal supplement, along with rest and a decrease in stress. Diet is also very important in treatment of the adrenals. Each time your blood sugars go low, it places an additional strain on the adrenal glands. This makes the hypoglycemic diet a priority.

In severe adrenal fatigue (a.k.a. poor adrenal reserve syndrome) I use low dose cortisone. This treatment is based on the work by Jefferies.* The principle behind this therapy is that we give a low dose of cortisone to supplement the adrenals. We keep this dose low so we do not turn the adrenals off. Cortisone has gotten a very bad reputation in this country because of how it has been used. If you take cortisone in high doses (that is doses that turn the adrenals off) for very long, it is almost certain that you will have side effects. Physicians in the U.S. usually prescribe cortisone in high doses, therefore, nearly everyone who takes it gets side-effects.

People forget that we make cortisone everyday. It is a natural product just like insulin or thyroid. If you do not make enough cortisone you will not function well. We produce roughly 40mg per day of cortisone. Our goal with this therapy is to supplement the adrenals, thereby allowing them to rest and hopefully regain their strength. In most people we use between 2.5 and 5.0mg of cortisone, two or three times a day.

Remember Prednisone is a synthetic cortisone which is four times stronger than cortisone. (5mg Prednisone is equal to 20mg

* Jefferies, William, Safe Uses of Cortisone, Thomas Books.

cortisone). One must be careful if using Prednisone, as you can shut off the adrenals with very low doses.

ACE: Adrenal Cortical Extract. This is used either sublingually or by IM (intramuscular injection). ACE is a natural product derived from ground cow adrenals, made into a sublingual solution or injection. The reason for using it this way is that cow adrenal extract taken by mouth is partially destroyed in the digestive tract. Using ACE sublingually or by IM injection bypasses that problem. ACE, when used as directed is very safe and I usually use this first before proceeding to low dose cortisone. I caution patients however that any natural treatment like ACE takes time*.

2. The Liver. The liver is perhaps the second hardest hit organ in chronic fatigue. Its ability to detoxify has been compromised. We approach this using several different methods. One is, we're careful to limit our use of medicines that are broken down in the liver. Drugs, such as Diflucan™ and Sporanox™ are broken down in the liver, therefore, we usually use short-term. If depression is severe, sometimes we will use an anti-depressant. We try to select the medicine that has the shortest half life (metabolized most quickly so that these medicines do not build up in the bloodstream). Often doctors become confused treating patients with chronic fatigue. They start these patients on what would be a normal dose for a normal adult and the patient often develops side effects. Many physicians inappropriately conclude that the patient is having a psychosomatic response. In reality these patients are not detoxifying well, therefore, normal doses of medications are to them the same as giving a normal person two or three times the normal dose. I tell the physicians that this is not unlike treating a senior citizen. When we have a senior citizen as a patient, we routinely start them off on a lower dose of medication than we would a young adult. The reason for this is that we assume that their liver and kidney function has diminished over time and, therefore, cannot detoxify the way a younger person can. However, because many patients with chronic fatigue appear on the outside to be normal, and the majority are younger than 50, doctors have a hard time comprehending that these patients cannot detoxify

---

* ACE is no longer available in the U.S.

the way a 'normal' person can. We also work at helping detoxification usually through use of supplements, modified fasting and the use of products designed to improve liver detoxification.

3.Thyroid. Low thyroid function is very common in patients with fatigue and chronic fatigue. Often this low thyroid function is not obvious. If it were obvious it would have been picked up by the many physicians these patients have seen before. This low thyroid function does not show up in the blood work. The blood work in the majority of instances appears normal. The reason for this is that thyroid blood work has such a wide range of normal. We do not have thyroid studies that are individualized for each person. Normal ranges on thyroid blood work are large, therefore, a person may very well have a sluggish thyroid and still fall within the ranges of normal on their blood work. It is then incorrectly assumed by their physician that their thyroid is normal. We have found this not to be the case. One reason for this is that many patients with fatigue are low in the amino acid tyrosine. A study conducted at the Fatigue Clinic of Michigan in 1994 showed that eighty-six percent of the CFIDS patients studied were low in the amino acids phenylalanine and tyrosine*. These deficiencies have tremendous implications. One problem is that several of the brain neurochemicals are made from tyrosine. These brain neurochemicals are called the catecholamines: norepinephrine and epinephrine. When tyrosine is low you have trouble making these normal brain chemicals. This is one of the factors that contributes to cognitive problems in chronic fatigue. Another problem is tyrosine is necessary for the production of thyroid hormone. Most people know that iodine is necessary for production of thyroid hormone, but they do not realize that the amino acid tyrosine, is also vital to make thyroxine. Tyrosine joins with iodine in the thyroid to produce thyroxine, (thyroxine is the normal thyroid hormone). Eighty-six percent of the patients in our study were low in tyrosine. This means that 86 percent of patients with CFIDS may have problems making normal thyroid hormone. Many times with the supplementation of tyrosine these patients are able to improve thyroid function. If their thyroid function does not improve with tyrosine, it may mean that their thyroid is sick. This may be due to inflammation of the thyroid

---

* Edward J. Conley *Amino Acid Deficiencies in Chronic Fatigue Syndrome, unpublished.*

(thyroiditis) in which case it may be necessary to use low doses of thyroid hormone. We might also add low doses of thyroid hormone if the patient's thyroid blood work was in the low normal ranges and they had many of the signs and symptoms consistent with hypothyroidism, along with low basal temperatures. Your basal temperature should be 97.6*. If it is lower than 97.6 consistently, it triggers us to be suspicious of a sluggish thyroid. We do not make the diagnosis solely on the low temperature, but we combine that with clinical signs and symptoms, patient history and lab studies. If necessary, we may also do a thyroid scan and uptake which tells us how well the thyroid is taking up iodine. Treatment of this subtle hypothyroidism is very important in the treatment of fatigue. One additional note about the thyroid, often times physicians will measure traditional thyroid lab studies. These appear to be normal, however, much of the thyroid hormone in the bloodstream may be bound to a protein called thyroid binding globulin (TBG). Once bound to TBG the thyroid hormone can't be used by the body. This gives a false reading of normal amounts of thyroid hormone when in reality much less free thyroid hormone is available to be used. So on a functional basis, the person is low thyroid even though their blood thyroid hormone levels appear normal. This can be corrected by the physician obtaining free thyroid hormone levels which are more expensive, but also more accurate. The free hormone levels give us a better picture of actually how much thyroid is available to be used. Also of importance is that many patients have a conversion defect of thyroid hormone, T4, to the more active hormone, T3. T3 is much more active than T4 and is the major active thyroid hormone in the body. T4 is made by the thyroid and then it is converted as needed to T3 by the body. Many people have trouble with this conversion. Often lab studies will show that patients are within normal on their free T4 but low in free T3.

If the physician did not measure the T3, they would not know this. Also, the most common thyroid replacement hormone in the United States is synthetic T4. It is assumed by physicians that this will be converted in the body to T3. I have seen many patients who have been on high doses of T4 thyroid replacement that were still functionally hypothyroid. The reason for this was that their bodies

---

* A basal temperature is taken for ten minutes first thing in the morning, before you get out of bed. Usually it's done under the arm (axillary).

were not able to convert the T4 they were being given to T3. Thyroid diagnosis and treatment can be confusing for physician and patient alike, and physicians in the United States need to take a more clinical approach to thyroid. The basic truth is that American doctors pay too much attention to blood work and not enough attention to the patient's clinical signs and symptoms!

# NUMBER FIVE:
## TREATMENT OF IMMUNE SYSTEM PROBLEMS AND ALLERGIES.

The vast majority of patients seen at our clinic with fatigue have multiple allergies. This includes allergies to foods, inhalants, dusts and pets. The diagnosis and elimination of these allergies is vital for the return to health. One commonly overlooked problem is food allergies. In nearly all patients seen for chronic fatigue we diagnose significant food allergies. It does not take a genius to figure out why. Almost all of these patients have bowel dysbiosis, which means the bowel itself is sick and allows larger molecules to pass into the bloodstream than is normal. (Please see Bowel Dysbiosis, chapter 9).

These patients are usually allergic to the foods that they eat most commonly. In the United States these foods are usually eggs, milk, wheat and corn. There is an old saying in allergy that you are mostly allergic to what you eat mostly, and this is very true for patients with fatigue. Elimination of these allergic foods and placing the patients on a rotation diet has given many people significant improvement both in fatigue and fibromyalgia. The nice thing about food allergies is that for the most part the patient can avoid them. (No expensive shots are necessary). This requires a special diet and patient determination to make this work. The bad thing about food allergies is that patients must do the work. There are extracts and injections for blocking food allergy reactions and sometimes we use them. However, for the most part, the mainstay of our treatment of food allergy is avoidance and use of the rotation diet. Avoidance is very important because we must stop the provocation of the immune system. The provocation of the immune system by allergic challenge is responsible for many of the signs and symptoms of chronic fatigue. (Either partially or completely). These include fibromyalgia, sinus drainage, sore throat, abdominal pain, cognitive dysfunction and asthma, just to name a few. Even more important, the continued provocation of the immune system will continue to put a drain on both the immune and adrenal systems. To control the inflammation as a result of the repeated allergic reactions, the body must produce cortisone. Cortisone is produced in the adrenals and if the adrenals are weak, forcing them to overwork will drain them further*. As I tell my patients it's as if you have a fractured foot and you keep stomping on it.

Identification and treatment of inhalant allergies are also important in chronic fatigue, if the inhalant allergy is severe, some form of neutralization therapy may be indicated. Usually I recommend provocation neutralization therapy as a way of more specifically identifying what dose of neutralization therapy is needed. An interesting form of treatment for allergies may be enzyme potentiated desensitization (EPD), which is currently being studied in the United States and in Europe. This may, indeed, be the next generation of treatment for allergy problems, although conclusive results are still pending. In any case, many times inhalant allergies are able to be controlled by avoidance. Usually we give patients detailed instructions on how to avoid the inhalants they are allergic to. It is important during the summer to keep the windows shut and to use air-conditioning, along with a proper HEPA air filtration system. Two of the toughest problems that we see in chronic fatigue are allergies to mold and dust mite. Allergy to mold is a huge problem. The vast majority of patients I see with fatigue are allergic to mold. Avoidance of mold is much more difficult because mold grows everywhere, including our homes. Mold counts are high if it's raining, or if leaves are wet and molding on the ground. Another problem is that mold is in foods. People with mold allergies seem to not only react to those foods that are moldy (including all foods that have been aged), but also to foods that have yeast in them. This includes beers, wines, yeast-risen breads, etc. This makes it hard for the patient to avoid mold, but it is possible. We council patients at length on the many ways of avoidance and treatment of mold allergy. One of the most

---

* The immune system is continually up regulated by the repeated challenge of food and inhalant allergens. This repeated activation of the immune system causes many symptoms and may lead to auto-immune disease where your own immune system starts to attack you.

important treatments of mold allergy is to decrease the yeast growing within you. To do this, please see our previous discussion on
restoring the ecosystem of the bowel (earlier in this chapter). Once
we reduce the overgrowth of yeast in the bowel, slowly the anti-yeast
antibodies, that are produced by the body in response to that
overgrowth, start to come down. This takes years, so once a person
is allergic to mold, it is reasonable to assume they will have that
allergy for many years. In addition to treatment of the internal
environment, we also treat the external environment. This includes
dehumidifiers in the basement, putting up a barrier between the
basement and the upper sections of the house, such as polyurethane
if the patient is not allergic to polyurethane. At times we may have to
block off the heating ducts and use electrical heat in the house.
Again, a HEPA filter is important and a good functional air-
conditioning system is essential. Please make sure that the air
conditioning system is clean, mold-free and filters changed frequently. (Nothing is worse than depending on your air-conditioner to
reduce the mold levels in your house and finding that the air-
conditioning unit itself is moldy). Dust mite allergy is also a severe
problem in those patients with chronic fatigue. Dust mite may be the
overall number one allergen in the United States. We are actually
allergic to the droppings from the dust mite. I read an incredible
statistic recently, if your pillow is more than a few years old, one-
tenth of its total weight consists of dust mites and dust mite droppings! This, of course, is something we snuggle our face up to for
eight hours every night and if you are allergic to dust mite, obviously
you've got problems in the morning. We work with our patients to
reduce the dust in their homes. This includes, where possible,
replacing old carpet with wood floors (which can be damp-mopped),
making sure all bedding is washed frequently in nontoxic detergent,
taking the mattress outside (if possible)—if it is below zero, this will
kill the dust mites, and removing collectibles from the bedroom. Also
available is barrier cloth which can seal you off from the dust mites in
your pillow and mattress.

## NUMBER SIX:
## TREATMENT OF COGNITIVE DYSFUNCTION.
Cognitive dysfunction is the second most common symptom

presented to me by fatigue patients. Fatigue, of course, being number one. Cognitive dysfunction takes place in up to 90 percent of fatigue patients. Many reasons for cognitive dysfunction have been proposed. It develops through a combination of circulatory, metabolic and neuroendocrine factors. The circulatory portion has been shown rather extensively. This has been demonstrated by special brain scans called SPECT scans. These SPECT scans show large areas of poor distribution of blood flow in many patients with CFS/CFIDS. The areas are usually pathognomonic for CFIDS (in most patients they occur in the same areas).

The exact reasons for these circulatory problems are currently unknown. However, one explanation may be that the brain fails to produce the proper chemicals, such as nitric oxide to allow for vascular dilatation. That is to say nitric oxide causes enlargement, or widening, of the vessels to the brain which would allow greater blood flow. Nitric oxide, by the way, is made from an amino acid. Remember, many patients with CFS/CFIDS are low in amino acids.

The second reason for cognitive dysfunction is inability of the brain to produce normal brain chemicals in the normal amounts. A study done at the Fatigue Clinic of Michigan (to be published) has shown that 86 percent of patients (who meet CDC criteria for chronic fatigue syndrome), were shown to be low in two of the amino acids that are necessary for production of normal brain chemicals. Those amino acids were phenylalanine and tyrosine. Phenylalanine and tyrosine are vital for making catecholamines, which are important in brain function. They are also necessary to make dopamine. Dopamine is vital in brain function as well. Without the proper amounts of phenylalanine and tyrosine the brain cannot make normal amounts of the brain chemicals dopamine and catecholamines and therefore function is diminished. Both of these brain substances are needed for normal nerve function. Tryptophan is the precursor to the brain chemical Serotonin. Serotonin is one of the brain chemicals that is necessary to prevent depression. The other brain chemicals norepinephrine and epinephrine as we've just discussed, are made from phenylalanine and tyrosine. So one thing is clear from this study, at least 85 percent of the patients with CFIDS/CFS we tested in this study were low in several essential amino acids. That means, more than likely, they were low in the brain chemicals that are made from those essential amino acids. This deficiency leads to difficulty with cognitive function and an actual physical reason for depression.

**IT IS IMPORTANT TO REALIZE JUST HOW IMPORTANT A POINT THAT LAST SENTENCE WAS. THERE IS AN ACTUAL PHYSIOLOGICAL REASON WHY PATIENTS WITH CHRONIC FATIGUE HAVE COGNITIVE DIFFICULTIES AND DEPRESSION!**

A third reason for cognitive dysfunction in fatigue is blood sugar fluctuations (hypoglycemia). At the Fatigue Clinic of Michigan we have found that the vast majority of patients with chronic fatigue have hypoglycemia. Hypoglycemia is the rapid fluctuation of blood sugar levels*. The brain runs on two main ingredients. Oxygen and glucose. Without those, the brain cannot function normally. When one or the other of these is low the brain will function abnormally. A very good example of this is when oxygen is diminished. When people go mountain-climbing and get above a certain point where the percentage of oxygen is reduced in the air, brain function becomes difficult, thinking is clouded, there are changes in moods and personality. This has been documented very extensively. What is also true, is that if you lower the other main ingredient that is necessary for brain function, glucose, the same things happens. That is to say, people get clouded thinking, personality changes and depression. I don't know why it is so hard for physicians to comprehend this. They know that if a person gets a decrease in oxygen, symptoms are certain, yet they deny that the same symptoms can result when you get changes in the second main ingredient needed for brain function, glucose. In people with chronic fatigue their blood sugars are bouncing around all throughout the day. When those blood sugars come down, they are going to have problems thinking. The exact time of hypoglycemia varies from patient to patient. Some patients have reactive hypoglycemia, which means that they can go two, three, four or five hours after eating and then the blood sugars drop precipitously. When those blood sugars drop, the patients have significant symptoms. Those symptoms include but are not limited to: clouded thinking, heart racing, sweating, personality changes,

---

* For the sake of this discussion we use glucose and sugar interchangeably. However, there are several types of sugar.

depression, irritation and fatigue. Another type of low blood sugar (hypoglycemia) is the low, flat curve. Those patients' blood sugars never really go up, nor do they drop precipitously at certain points. They seem to have a slow downward slope, but still they respond with symptoms like those with reactive hypoglycemia. Those of you with blood sugar fluctuations, will have thinking problems and personality changes. (The brain operates within set parameters just like the engine of a car. If you get the fuel of an automobile out of certain parameters, the engine will not run right or may even stall. With the brain, if you get the fuel, which is glucose, out of parameters, the brain will not function right). How do we treat cognitive changes? We do that by treating their causes.

**Cognitive Treatment Number One:** We address the deficiencies of amino acids. It is clear from my research that at least 85 percent of the patients with chronic fatigue have amino acid deficiencies and it is reasonable to assume that those amino acid deficiencies are causing deficiencies in the appropriate brain chemicals. What we do is identify those deficiencies and supplement with the proper amino acids to correct them. Why so many people are low in phenylalanine, tyrosine and tryptophan in unknown. It could be for several reasons: 1) Those amino acids called aromatic amines need the proper pH in the stomach to be digested. One important reason why you are not digesting those amino acids is lack of stomach acid. There have been many studies done which show that a large percentage of Americans are hypochlorhydric. That means that they are low in stomach acid. This causes the pH in the stomach to be too high. An additional reason for low stomach acid may be the over-use of H2 blockers in this country. H2 blockers are medicines, such as Tagamet™, Zantac™, Pepcid™, Prilosec™ and Axid™. Those medications reduce the secretion of acid in the stomach, thereby increasing the stomach pH. (I have a big concern that this problem will become worse as now these H2 blockers are over-the-counter, and can be used by anyone who has 'acid indigestion', without a prescription). In reality, their indigestion may not be caused by the overproduction of acid, but by the underproduction of acid or by food allergies! However, that's a topic of a whole separate book. In any case, proper supplementation of the amino acids are necessary and correction of

155

the acid balance of the stomach is essential. We supplement the amino acid, tyrosine, if it is deficient. Tyrosine has a stimulatory effect, so we do not give tyrosine in the evening\*. Tryptophan is not available over-the-counter in the United States, having been withdrawn by the Food and Drug Administration. It is available by prescription in the form of L-Tryptophan, which you must obtain from your physician[†]. Tryptophan is also available in foods that we eat. I recommend to patients with sleep difficulties to increase their Tryptophan foods in the evening. These foods include: low fat milk, turkey, yogurt and soy beans. (Please make sure you are not allergic to these foods prior to increasing their use).

## Cognitive Treatment Number Two:

We use several medications designed to improve the blood flow to the brain or improve how the brain utilizes oxygen. One of those is called <u>Ginkgo</u>. Ginkgo is actually an herb that has been used for thousands of years in the Orient to improve mental function. It is the most commonly used medicine in the Orient for senile dementia (which is commonly referred to as hardening of the arteries). The reason for this is that Ginkgo is a mild vasodilator of the cerebral vasculature. That means that Ginkgo causes some widening of the arteries that supply the brain with blood. This widening of the arteries allows more blood to the brain, therefore more oxygen and more nutrients. The only side effect that we have seen with Ginkgo is headache (cephalalgia)\*\*. If headache ensues then you need to reduce the dose of the medication. Headaches are usually dose-dependent. You must be careful as sometimes the headaches can be insidious and if you have recurrent headaches do not automatically think that you're having migraines, you must consider reducing the Ginkgo.

## Treatment Medication Number One: Hydergine™.

Hydergine™ is a prescription medication available in the United States that contains ergoloid and mesylates. It is believed that

---

\* Tyrosine can trigger migraines in susceptible individuals. Also, if you are on a MAO inhibitor <u>do not</u> take Tyrosine. Consult a physician prior to use.
[†] L-Tryptophan is now available by prescription only in the U.S.
\*\* The headache resolves by reducing the dose.

these substances improve how the brain utilizes oxygen. This medication does not improve the blood flow to the brain, but may improve how the brain utilizes the oxygen that it gets. This medicine does not have a good reputation for effectiveness in the United States. However, it is highly regarded in Europe.

The reason for this difference may lie in the fact that the European dose is considerably higher than the American dose. The European dose is roughly three times as strong as the American dose. I have found a significant number of patients with chronic fatigue get some improvement from a dose of two or three tablets, three times daily. Hydergine™ has virtually no side effects. Transient nausea and gastric disturbances have been reported but the PDR states that Hydergine™ preparations have not been found to produce serious side effects. Therefore, except for the expense involved, these medications are good to try for the cognitive problems in chronic fatigue. Often times we combine therapies such as combining Ginkgo and Hydergine along with choline.

## Cognitive Treatment Number Three: Choline.

Choline is important to make the brain chemical acetylcholine. Acetylcholine is necessary for nerve function. Most people think that nerves are hooked together like extension cords, that they plug into each other, but this is not true. Nerves do not hook into each other. They do not meet. There is a small area between nerves called the synapse. What happens is when a nerve is stimulated it produces acetylcholine with a certain message. That acetylcholine goes into the synapse, is picked up by the appropriate nerve on the other end of the synapse and the message continues to be sent. This allows our nerves to function very quickly. Otherwise, if we had nerves that all hooked into each other, it would take us all day to add two plus two. This way, one nerve can fire and trigger millions of other nerves which then fire and trigger billions of other nerves, all in a microsecond. However, if you are low in acetylcholine it may diminish the efficiency of how those nerves fire and how the messages are transmitted. Choline is a substance which we should derive from our food. You can think of it as being part of the Vitamin B family, at least it is usually considered along with the B vitamins. Many patients with fatigue seen at FCM are low in choline. Choline

157

has become a very popular treatment for senile dementia (declining mental function of senior citizens), in Europe and the Orient. Choline can be obtained over-the-counter at your local health food store. It can be taken in several ways, one is choline cocktail which comes in powder form. The powder, you mix into a drink. Another form can be obtained more cheaply by supplementing with phosphatidyl choline. Phosphatidyl choline is made from soybeans, (soybeans are high in choline). An even cheaper source of choline is to take soybean lecithin daily.

## Cognitive Treatment Number Four: DHEA.

DHEA, we have discussed at length in chapter 14. There is a large amount of research currently underway on DHEA effects on Alzheimer's disease and cognitive function. It has been shown that patients with Alzheimer's disease are lower in DHEA than patients without Alzheimer's disease. We know that DHEA improves cellular energy production, and that DHEA enhances immunity. It may be by this improvement in cellular energy production that cognitive function is improved. We only use DHEA if you are shown to be deficient in DHEA by blood and urine studies. When you combine the above medications along with supplementation of deficient amino acids in conjunction with our overall treatment program for improving chronic fatigue syndrome, you will have improvement in your cognitive function. The vast majority of patients at FCM have had improvement in their cognitive state. It is important to remember, however, that these improvements take time, usually months.

## Cognitive Treatment Number Five: Serotonin Reuptake Inhibitors.

This class includes: Prozac™, Zoloft™, Paxil™, Effexor™, and Serzone™. These are medications which have received a large amount of news coverage over the last five years. Basically they work by slowing down the breakdown of Serotonin in the brain. As we've already discussed, serotonin is one of the major anti-depression brain chemicals. There are two ways that you can improve serotonin. One is to make more, the other is to decrease how much is being broken down. We have already reviewed with you how to make more by increasing the amount of tryptophan. The pharmaceutical industry has come up with the second way, and that is by reducing the re-uptake of serotonin. This means they have reduced the breakdown of serotonin which leads to increased amounts of serotonin in the brain. I have no problem with using this therapy except for the following facts: 1) it is expensive; 2) there are side effects; and 3) you may have to be on the medication for the rest of your life. The reason for this is that this medication does not fix anything. It simply reduces the breakdown of serotonin. If you stop the medicine your serotonin levels drop. At our clinic we use this medication for those people who are significantly depressed and whom we're concerned about the depression causing them to commit suicide. We use these medications when a quick treatment is needed. The natural therapies are excellent as long as we have time to let them work. However, if I am concerned about a patient hurting themselves, I will use these anti-depressant medications. I always try and look at these as short-term medicines, not a long-term solution.

**Cognitive Treatment Number Six: Hormone Therapy.**
      Almost all patients with fatigue have hormone deficiencies. Hormones are produced by a system we call the endocrine system. That system includes: the pituitary gland in the brain which gets its instructions from the hypothalamus (which is part of the brain). The system also includes the thyroid, pancreas, adrenals, testicles, ovaries and the parathyroid glands. These glands are responsible for the production of hormones which have many responsibilities in the body. Deficiencies in patients with fatigue include the following (not all patients have deficiencies of all of these hormones, however, many patients have multiple deficiencies as discussed below):

A. DHEA (Please see chapter 14) DHEA is a hormone that's produced by the adrenals and is named the 'mother hormone'. It's named the 'mother hormone' because DHEA can be converted by the body into multiple other hormones. It used to be thought that DHEA was only an intermediate hormone, that is, something that was just around to be made into another hormone. However, we now know that DHEA is important in and of itself, both for immunity and energy production. How does DHEA become low, and why is it low in patients with fatigue and CFS? There are multiple reasons why this occurs:

1. We know that DHEA diminishes as we age. The reasons for this are not altogether clear except in general, adrenal function appears to diminish as we age. This may account for the decrease in immunity and energy production as we age and follows a general trend of diminishment of the endocrine system's production of hormones as we age.

2. Another important factor and, indeed, perhaps the most important factor is that DHEA is diminished due to stress. (See page 54). DHEA is usually made from the precursor hormone pregnenolone in the adrenals. In times of stress, however, we have an alternative pathway that allows the adrenals to divert pregnenolone from DHEA and make it into cortisol. Cortisol being the more important hormone when we are under stress. This has survival advantages which I explained in Chapter 14. This is much like the analogy of when we are at war; we convert our automobile plants to tank plants, tanks being the priority. However, with our stresses these days being long-term stresses, we follow what's called the Pregnenolone steal pathway or the increased conversion of pregnenolone to cortisol for long periods of time. This causes a decrease in circulating DHEA. As DHEA decreases, so does overall immunity and our ability to produce energy. This I suspect, along with nutritional deficiencies, is by far the most common reason why patients with chronic fatigue are low in DHEA. We evaluate patients for DHEA insufficiency both by blood and urine evaluation. If patients are low in DHEA, they're easily treated by supplementing DHEA either by pill or by cream (topical). At our clinic we use DHEA in small doses and we monitor both DHEA levels and liver function studies carefully every three months. We have been able to use DHEA in conjunction with our total treatment program very successfully. DHEA, however, is not without possible side effects and should not be used lightly. In the proper hands, I feel DHEA is a very good treatment for CFS,* if used, as stated above, in conjunction with a total treatment program. DHEA by itself is not the answer to chronic fatigue.

B. Cortisone. As strange as it may seem, given the discussion

---

* Only use DHEA if you are low in DHEA and only with a physician's supervision.

above, many patients actually appear to be low in cortisone. This develops for several reasons. The adrenals overall appear to be worn down in chronic fatigue. The progression of the wearing down of the adrenals goes something like this. In the beginning, the adrenals are called on to work more often and are able to hold up to the task for the first few months, or in those who are strong for the first few years. However, eventually the adrenals start to wear down. As they become tired they allow our sugars to fluctuate more wildly. Eventually, through continued stress, nutritional deficiency, fluctuations in blood sugars and possibly neuroendocrine problems (that is to say, trouble with the brain producing cortical-stimulating hormone) the adrenals become worn down. Once they become worn down a person cannot handle stress. They have difficulty maintaining adequate blood sugars and therefore have hypoglycemic events. They feel overall muscle weakness and fatigue. This may happen without many of the lab findings associated with severe cortisone deficiency, something named Addison's disease. Addison's disease is a disease associated with a severe low output state of the adrenals. This results in severe fatigue, muscle weakness, bronzing of the skin and sugar fluctuations. What we usually see with CFS is a less severe form of adrenal fatigue called poor adrenal reserve. If a person is at a point where their adrenals are stressed but their adrenal function appears to be adequate most of the time, the key is to reduce the stress, correct nutritional deficiencies and give the adrenals some support. This support is usually in the form of nutrients that are important for the adrenals. It may also include some adrenal supplementation. At our clinic this usually takes the form of adrenal extracts. Adrenal extracts are ground adrenal, usually of cow origin (bovine). This is taken to help support the person's adrenals, along with a total program of increased rest, decreased stress, appropriate nutrition and nutritional supplements. If the adrenals have gone beyond mild fatigue and have entered into severe fatigue, they require more aggressive treatment. Usually that consists of rest, proper nutrition and nutritional supplements, but also the use of adrenal cortical extracts (ACE). ACE is a form of adrenal which more aggressively supplements and stabilizes the adrenals*. Adrenal Cortical Extract is exactly what is says, an extract of cow adrenal. It does

* ACE is currently unavailable in the United States

contain very small amounts of cortisone which usually scares people. Remember that we produce around 40mg of cortisone daily and without it we would be dead. If you are not able to produce cortisone properly, you cannot be healthy. It is the overuse of cortisone that is a danger. While the use of any adrenal extract or supplement is to be used with caution, it is no where near as dangerous as the commonplace use of high doses of cortisone prescribed by traditional practitioners. These high doses of cortisone (either oral or injectable) almost always turn off the adrenal glands. When that happens you are always assured of side effects. Our goal is not to turn off the adrenals but simply to supplement them. These extracts are usually used without side effect. Indeed, many of our patients have had significant symptomatic improvement by the use of these extracts. They've been able to stabilize both their loss of strength and the fluctuations of their blood sugars. Another form of adrenal supplement is to use small doses of cortisone several times a day as has be proposed by Jeffries. This therapy we reserve for those with more severe adrenal fatigue. We will always use the less aggressive therapy of adrenal supplements first. If the patient doesn't improve we consider low dose cortisone. Combined with all the treatments that we've talked about in this chapter and throughout the book, these adrenal regimens have proven to be an excellent treatment for chronic fatigue.

C. Melatonin. Melatonin is a hormone that is produced by our pineal gland. The pineal is a small gland in the brain that produces both melatonin and serotonin. Melatonin is responsible for allowing us to go to sleep naturally. It also has other functions which are now starting to come to light, such as it appears to be an extraordinarily good antioxidant. Melatonin is a small molecule that defuses easily and appears to cross every internal barrier, including the blood brain barrier. Furthermore, experiments in Italy (at the National Institute for Research on Aging, in Ancona, Italy), have shown that melatonin can counteract the shrinkage of the thymus gland. The thymus gland is important for producing T-cells, which are an important part of our immune system. There is currently a tremendous amount of research proceeding on the effects of melatonin in the human body. In my experience, there are many patients in which melatonin is helpful for establishing a more normal sleep cycle. Indeed, the lack of, or deficiency in melatonin may be one of the major reasons why the sleep cycle becomes disturbed in patients with chronic fatigue. How does his happen? Melatonin is decreased due to stress. As we've pointed out before, not only have we found that patients with chronic fatigue had a large amount of stressors in their past, but development of fatigue itself adds to the stress. This may cause a downward spiral where the more stress, the worsening of the Melatonin deficiency, the worsening of our sleep disturbances, the more fatigue, and so on. Melatonin appears to be an important hormonal deficiency in chronic fatigue. This is one that is easily addressed. I recommend melatonin for patients with sleep disturbances. Usually we proceed with melatonin 3 to 6mg at bedtime, actually one hour prior to bedtime. Not only does this help the sleep disturbances, but it is also a very good antioxidant which people with chronic fatigue need. Since oxidative damage is major problem in chronic fatigue syndrome, antioxidants such as melatonin, maybe very beneficial in stabilizing the oxidative damage. For a complete discussion of oxidative damage in chronic fatigue, please see *The Canary and Chronic Fatigue*, by Majid Ali, M.D. Melatonin helps to restore normal sleep cycles but you must be cautioned that it can take some time. Often we have to use it in combination with other natural therapies and at times we use it in combination with prescription medications. I try to look at the prescription medications as being a temporary treatment. The long-term treatment is reestablishing the normal mechanism of how you fall asleep. Let's review briefly how melatonin is produced and how it enables us to fall asleep naturally. What happens is, as it becomes dark our brain senses the amount of light in the ambient surroundings. As dusk and then darkness comes on, our brain starts to produce melatonin. Melatonin then slowly increases through the evening where it reaches its highest point before midnight. (This is true for those people who are not on third shift). Light can disturb our production of melatonin. As I stated above, it is the recognition of the darkness that starts the melatonin production. Melatonin can be affected by artificial light. That is to say, if you leave all the lights in your house on and then you abruptly turn them off and want to go straight to bed and go to sleep, you may have a problem. The problem is that your body does not function that way. Most people do not understand the mechanism of how we fall asleep. It's that our body must recognize darkness and after we've recognized darkness then we produce melatonin. It takes several hours of melatonin production to get us ready for sleep. That is why I counsel my patients that at an appropriate time of night, at least one hour prior to bedtime, they should turn off their artificial lights. If someone in the family must read, then I ask that they read by a small reading light or book light. Also turn off other sources of light, such as the television. If someone must watch television, they should do so away from the patient with chronic fatigue. This allows the patient with chronic fatigue to be exposed to darkness and allows the brain to adjust the time clock by production of melatonin. As trivial as this may seem, this is an important point in treatment of sleep disturbances. There is something called light pollution and basically what this means is that during the night it is very easy for us to snap on lights and expose our brain to rather strong concentration of artificial daylight. This has been called light pollution. We recommend to patients that if they have to get up in the night, that they not turn on the lights, that they have low level night lights available so that they're able to get up and navigate to the bathroom, etc., without exposing their brain to large amounts of light. Again, this is something that you wouldn't ordinarily think about, but it is an important factor for those people with sleep disturbances.

D. Testosterone. Something unusual has been happening with the testosterone levels of men in the United States. First of all, let me state that testosterone is usually thought of as being important only for men, that's it a male hormone and that it's only important in giving men their hair and sex drive. However, testosterone is important for women and men. The difference being, of course, that men have more testosterone than women. Testosterone, however, is far more important than just giving people their sex drive. Testosterone is vital for energy production and muscle strength. The building up of muscle is what we call an anabolic state. Testosterone also gives us a feeling of well being. What is anabolic state? The body can exist in two different modes. Anabolic, which means building up or catabolic, which means tearing down. Testosterone is one of the anabolic hormones. This means that with proper amounts of testosterone and a proper diet, your body stays in positive nitrogen balance and this allows you to maintain and/or build muscle. Testosterone also allows us to produce the energy that's necessary for using that muscle. Catabolism is the process of tearing down. When the body is in a catabolic state it means that it does not have the nutrients available and/or the anabolic hormones necessary to keep it from tearing itself down. One important example of this is when you do not get the quality protein that you need on a daily basis, your body will go into negative nitrogen balance and your body will start to tear down your own muscles for the amino acids that are necessary for day to day operation. If you stay in the catabolic state long enough, it will cause you to become weaker, resulting in the loss of muscle strength and size. Testosterone is important in keeping both men and women in the anabolic camp. That is to say on the side of building up and not on the side of tearing down. Now, why do I say there's something strange going on with testosterone in the United States? In the past, low testosterones have been associated with men 50 to 70 years of age. However, it is now starting to be seen that men even in their 30's and 40's are low in testosterone. This is resulting in decreased muscle strength, endurance and production of sperm. (A scary statistic is that an adult male now produces one-half as much sperm as an adult male did in 1929). There may be several reasons for the decreased levels of testosterone. It has been hypothesized that part of the reason is pollution. Many of the chemical pollutants produced resemble estrogen. When these chemicals are ingested by the male, they act as an estrogenic force in the body causing the relative ratio of testosterone to estrogen to decline. This certainly may be an important part of the decrease in sperm production and cannot be underestimated. Another important reason, and I think the dominant problem, is <u>stress</u>. I believe that stress is causing a large percentage of the loss of production of testosterone. How does this happen? Testosterone is produced from DHEA. DHEA is produced from pregnenolone. As we discussed in both the DHEA chapter and earlier in this chapter, when you are under stress you body shunts pregnenolone to the production of cortisol and away from the production of DHEA. With the dropping levels of DHEA, you start to get drops in the levels of testosterone. This, of course, eventually leads to low circulating testosterone and to many of the symptoms listed earlier. An additional problem appears to be that there is a reduction in circulation of free testosterone in the body. A hormone can circulate in two possible ways. One is bound. That means where the hormone is bound to a protein and the other is unbound, or free. It is this free hormone that is available for use by the body. The bound hormone, because it is bound to another protein, is used with difficulty and most of the time cannot be used. There is evidence that there are decreases in the amount of testosterone that is circulating as free testosterone and increases in the amount of testosterone circulating as bound testosterone. Exactly why this is happening is unclear. Again, speculation abounds that perhaps this is because of chemical pollutants. Several chemicals are able to attach to the testosterone molecule and not allow its use. There may be an autoimmune phenomenon involved (the body attacking its own hormones), although this is unclear. This is the reason why at our clinic we measure free testosterone levels along with total testosterone levels. One thing is clear for men, and that is that we are reaching 'male menopause' at a much earlier age than in times past. This is something that is virtually ignored by modern medicine and yet is a source of significant symptoms in the adult male population. As we've already mentioned, these symptoms include: fatigue, depression, muscle weakness, decreases in immunity, lower sex drive and poor sperm production. It is so foolish for doctors to think that these patients are merely depressed. I suppose women can feel that at last men are finally getting their own since for years and years doctors have told women that they were just depressed when undergoing the hormonal changes in menopause. However, as women will gladly attest, these hormonal changes cause significant physiological problems and symptoms which are not psychosomatic! It is time for the doctors in the United States to realize the important function that hormones play in normal health, and the problems that are created when those hormones are out of balance or deficient. This is a shame since testosterone is so easily replaced. Once you have identified that there is a deficiency in testosterone, there are various ways of replacement. One is the old form, which is replacement by injection. Newer forms have now been developed where testosterone is able to be replaced by a testosterone patch or cream, both applied to the scrotum daily. All of these therapies are relatively low cost, and if used properly are relatively low in possible side effects. They give dramatic improvement for those patients who are low in testosterone. Usually, however, we have to combine many therapies for endocrine dysfunction. That is to say, it is not uncommon to see a person who is clinically low in cortisone, DHEA and testosterone. We must supplement all of these carefully if we are to improve the condition. We will talk more about that at the end of this chapter.

E. <u>Progesterone.</u> Progesterone is important in females for regulation of the menstrual periods and controlling premenstrual syndrome, among other functions. If you refer the diagram on page 54, the Pregnenolone Steal Pathway, you will see that progesterone is made from pregnenolone. If pregnenolone is being taken and converted to cortisol by the Pregnenolone steal pathway, it is not being converted to progesterone. This happens because of stress, usually prolonged stress. As this happens a woman will get decreased production of progesterone which may lead to menstrual abnormalities and increasing premenstrual symptoms. It is important that these deficiencies be identified and treated. If you just treat the progesterone deficiency, you have improved the situation but you've not optimally treated the patient. For those women who are low in progesterone, I suspect strongly they also have some adrenal fatigue and we must evaluate their DHEA, cortisol and progesterone levels and treat accordingly. Because the endocrine system is interrelated it is not uncommon to see deficiencies of several of the hormones that are produced by the endocrine system. Supplementation in an attempt to balance this system is vital for re-energizing the person with fatigue. This, in combination with the improvement in energy production that results by treating the blocks in the Krebs cycle, forms the back bone for an effective treatment program for fatigue and CFIDS/CFS.

## Cognitive Treatment Number Seven: Diet and Exercise.

The importance of diet in the treatment of fatigue cannot be overestimated. Not only is it important to know what to eat, but it's just as important to know what to avoid. We usually start with teaching people the basics, and that is we have them use fresh, clean foods. By that, we mean avoidance of as much pesticides and herbicides as possible and avoidance of antibiotics. Most animal foods, such as milk or meat, will contain antibiotics. The reason for this is that most poultry and livestock are routinely fed antibiotics to prevent them from getting infections. Milk cattle are fed antibiotics routinely for the same reason. These antibiotics then show up in the meat and milk that we eat and drink. (Therefore if we're not careful, we end up getting small doses of antibiotic on a daily basis, even though we are not taking any antibiotics ourselves). Even these small doses of antibiotics can further decrease our normal bacteria and produce a worsening of the overgrowth of yeast or abnormal 'bad' (pathogenic) bacteria. This in spite of the fact that you have been careful not to over use antibiotics for your personal use. The best situation would be to use organic food which often can be purchased from cooperatives or from health food stores. You may also inquire of organic gardening clubs in your area to see if any of them sell their produce. However, organic food is not always available and it is more costly. You may then want to use clean food. By clean food I mean it is grown by farmers who have not routinely given the animals antibiotics, or have not routinely sprayed their crops with pesticides or herbicides, but yet whose land is not certified organic. You may do this by utilizing farmers' markets where you get an opportunity to talk with the farmers who actually raise the produce. Or find farmers in your area that you can work with. You may also want to form a cooperative among your support groups or friends where you can speak with farmers who will raise produce specifically for your club. In any case, get his done because the antibiotics, as I've already explained, reduce your good bacteria further. The pesticides and herbicides work to damage your enzymes that are important in energy production. Therefore, the avoidance of both of these are important. Secondly, avoidance of those foods to which you are allergic is vital. I also recommend that patients avoid those foods that contain mold or yeast. We used to wait for the laboratory studies to be completed, but since our studies have shown that almost 90 percent of my patients with chronic fatigue have allergies to mold, and since it is one of the most common allergies in the United States, we automatically recommend an anti-yeast diet. This is also known as the anti-candida diet. For an in-depth discussion of the anti-candida diet, please see *The Yeast Connection Handbook* by Dr. William Crook (See Addendum II). Basically what an anti-candida diet is, is avoidance of those foods that are high in mold or yeast and avoidance of those foods that are high in sugar. The foods that are high in mold and yeast include, but are not limited to, beers and wines, aged cheeses, fermented products, aged or dried meats or fruits, mushroom products and yeast-risen products. Also, where possible, avoidance of canned products in favor of frozen or fresh. For complete discussion of this, please see the chapter on candida. Avoidance of these foods are important so you do not continue to trigger allergic reactions by exposing yourself to mold and yeast. We also recommend strongly a basic hypoglycemia diet. The reason we recommend this is because so many people have fluctuations in their blood sugar, otherwise known as low blood sugar (hypoglycemia). This diet is quite simple. Basically, it means avoidance of all sweets (as much as possible), and making sure that you do not go too long without eating. You must experiment with this and find out what schedule is best for you. Some people have to eat very small amounts every two hours, others are able to stick with their usual meal schedule as long as they do not skip meals. In general, I recommend you have small meals at breakfast, lunch and dinner, and to have in-between snacks mid-morning and mid-afternoon, and if need be, before bed. The way that you'll know if you need a snack before bed is if you find yourself waking up at the same time every night. For instance, if you wake up at 3 a.m. every morning, this should be a clue to you that you may be having a low blood sugar reaction in the middle of the night and you should have a small snack at bedtime. The hypoglycemia diet is important so you can stop the wild fluctuations in blood sugar. Controlling your blood sugar will help your adrenals to recover faster. Not only that, but it will help decrease some symptoms, such as: cloudy thinking, acute episodes of fatigue, sweatiness and palpitations of the heart, just to name a few. For a complete discussion of this please see the chapter on hypoglycemia (Chapter 11). Remember to adjust your diet, eating fresh, clean foods and avoid those foods that you are allergic to. Also avoid those foods that are high in mold, and follow a basic hypoglycemia diet. Adjusting your diet is just as important as the medicines that we prescribe!

Exercise. Perhaps the question asked most often in my office is how much should I exercise and what type of exercise should I do? My basic answer to patients with severe fatigue and chronic fatigue syndrome is that first of all exercise should <u>not</u> cause you to have post-exertional fatigue. By that I mean, if you exercise and the next day you feel worse, you have overdone it. You must be very careful with aerobic exercise. Aerobic exercise includes bike-riding, walking, swimming, running or anything that gets the heart rate up. The reason for this is that people with severe fatigue or chronic fatigue syndrome tolerate aerobic exercise poorly. The reason for this is that the enzymes of the Krebs cycle have been damaged. Remember that the Krebs cycle is how we generate energy aerobically. If the Krebs cycle is not functioning as well as it should, we cannot generate energy for aerobic exercise as well as we should. Therefore, aerobic exercise should be done with extreme caution. You should start off very slowly and you should increase very slowly, preferably exercising every other day. This allows your body some time to recover and rebuild energy. For those people with fatigue problems that seem to improve with exercise, you can increase the aerobic exercise more quickly. The only way you would know this is through experimentation and again I caution you to start off <u>very carefully</u>!

Most patients with CFS/CFIDS tolerate anaerobic exercise much better than aerobic exercise. What anaerobic exercise means is that it does not increase the heart rate to a significant degree. One fine example of an anaerobic exercise is weight-lifting. Most patients with CFIDS are able to tolerate weight-lifting. Again, we caution them to start off with very light weights and to do it every other day. Weight-lifting of course does several things: 1) it helps the patient maintain muscle tone and muscle strength, in spite of the fact that they are not able to be active. 2) it allows for some increased circulation to the muscles; 3) it allows the patient to do some exercise which causes an increased production of endorphins. Endorphins are the natural painkilling substances in your brain. (The positive effects of weight-lifting have been well documented in nearly all age groups. I recommend you begin a weight-lifting program every other day, starting at extremely light weights. If you are a woman, you may even want to start with a one pound weight doing whatever number of repetitions you can tolerate comfortably. If you are a man, you may start at between five and ten pounds, again at whatever repetitions you can tolerate comfortably and then stop. Try to work your arms and legs. To work your legs you may need to buy some inexpensive leg weights, and do some straight-leg raises. These can be done with or without weights. See how you feel the next day. If you feel good, continue to lift at this weight for at least two weeks before slowly increasing your weight. Again, I caution you, do not increase your weight too much or too quickly. Take your time because we want you to stay with weight-lifting exercise indefinitely.

## SUMMARY

1. Chronic fatigue and CFS/CFIDS are not caused by a single factor. Nor will it be resolved by a single treatment. To wait for a single treatment (i.e. drug) is foolish, even if one were to develop (which I doubt) it will take years to come on the market.

2. You can get better! Progress will be slow, you have not been sick for three months, you will not get better in three months. Nearly everyone who follows this program improves. Most get 50%+ improvement. Many return to normal function. I cannot tell you how long it will take, how much therapy you will require or how much better you will get. All I can tell you is that you will improve.

3. To improve you must follow the whole program. Some parts do not apply to everyone—and when that happens, obviously you don't have to adhere to them. Overall, however, you must be evaluated for all the components and treated accordingly. Remember, the goal of this program is to restore you to health—not fight a disease. These may sound the same, but they mean two entirely different things. For instance, we can give you a medicine to help 'fight' your viral infection and you might feel better. However if we leave it at that you will eventually become sick again. Why? Because you have not resolved any of the underlying problems that caused you to 'come down' with the virus in the first place. We must remember always to treat the <u>problem</u>, not the <u>symptom</u>!

4. You will have set-backs. No one gets better exponentially . Almost everyone gets better in a way that resembles stair steps. So you will

171

have periods of time where you will hit plateaus. Accept them and look for ways to elevate yourself to the next level. It's a process not unlike unloading many bales of straw off a camel's back—you just keep unloading as you find the bales because you never know which one will finally allow the camel to get back on its feet. All the bales of straw that came before are of equal importance, not just the 'one that broke the camel's back'.

5. Find a specialist in chronic fatigue. Preferably one that under-stands that you must be restored to health. You will waste more time and <u>far</u> more money by working with a physician that doesn't understand the principles of fatigue. Even though physicians who specialize in fatigue are more costly in the short-term they will save you thousands of dollars in the long run. Example: If you are delayed in getting back to work by three years, the cost would be $40,000X3 =$120,000! Not to mention the personal cost to you and your family during that time.

6. Use the power at your disposal. If you are religious, pray. Remem-ber God can do anything. Also remember that not all prayers are answered immediately. The right set of circumstances must be in place. Perhaps you reading this is part of the answer to your prayer. If you are not religious then meditate daily. There is tremendous power in the Universe. Through meditation you can tap into this power. Use your 'gut' feeling. Let it direct your actions. Through meditation you can quiet the noise and discover what your 'gut' feelings are. Those feelings come from the heart and the heart is seldom wrong. (For a resource on this you may review the works of Deepak Chopra, M.D.). Autoregulation as described by Majid Ali, M.D. is an effective way of quieting your mind so that your body can start to heal.

     <u>Above all else, never quit—never give up!</u> There is a big difference between accepting your current limitations and working within them, all the while realizing that you will eventually get better, versus accepting the 'fact' that you will be like this the rest of your life. When in reality you <u>don't</u> have to be like this the rest of your life. Don't let any doctor tell you that there is nothing you can do! You now know, there is <u>everything</u> you can do.

Remember, every journey begins with a first step. Please take that first step and the steps after that. Don't wait—your health is too important to wait. Your health and the health of your loved ones is your most important asset. Far more important than money, status or job. I have several millionaires as patients who would tell you that.

So get started—seek out a fatigue specialist, evoke the power of the Universe and never give up!

I wish you Godspeed on this journey and I hope the information in this book will help guide your way.

With Best Wishes,
Dr. Edward J. Conley

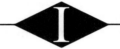

## ADDENDUM

# WHAT ELSE IS INEXPENSIVE AND POSSIBLY HELPFUL?

Make your bedroom more environmentally-safe and allergy-free.

1. Clean it from top to bottom with Shaklee cleaning products.

2. Put pure cotton towels in a 100% cotton pillow case.

3. Cover your mattress with a pad made from heavy-duty freezer aluminum foil, the shiny side up. Or, use a barrier cloth.

4. Use a quality air purifier if you can afford one. This might cost $200 to $300 but sometimes you can sleep with less congestion or asthma and awaken happy and content. (Call PARF (716) 875-0398).

5. Try to eliminate molds in the family bathroom and basement. Use Shaklee Basic G (check phone book for local distributors) to clean these areas. Use Bon Ami polishing powder to replace odorous scouring powder.

6. Stop all scented items, aerosols and chemical-smelling personal or cleaning preparations in your home (particularly in the bedroom and bathroom).

7. Compare how you feel, act, behave, your pulse, your breathing, your writing and your drawing before and 10 to 40 minutes after you eat or drink, go into every room at home/school/work, go outside versus inside, smell an unavoidable chemical or engage in your hobby. If you feel, act, or behave worse in some way, your pulse increases by 20, your breathing (peak Flow Meter) drops by 20%, or your writing or drawing is worse, find out what you ate, touched or smelled that is a problem.

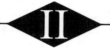

**ADDENDUM**

# Anti-Candida Diet

*The following Anti-Candida diet is excerpted from The Yeast Connection Handbook by William G. Crook, M.D. Professional Books Inc. and printed with permission. To order this or any of Dr. Crook's work call 1-800-227-2627.*

Your next step is diet. Compare what you'd need to do if you were taking a three-week ocean voyage on a sailing ship. Before you start your trip you'd have to get enough food. I'm not asking you to buy *all* of it and store it in your pantry and refrigerator, yet here are my suggestions for getting started:

Go to your kitchen, pantry and refrigerator and get rid of the sugar, corn syrup, white bread and other white flour products, soda pop, most ready to eat cereals, and all the sweet, fat snack foods. *Foods and beverages containing these nutritionally deficient simple carbohydrates encourage yeast overgrowth and promote poor health.* To overcome your candida related health problems you'll need to avoid them.

Replace them with more vegetables of all kinds, including some that you may not usually eat. Also go to the health food store and buy the grain alternatives, including amaranth, buckwheat and quinoa. (You'll find instructions for preparing and serving them in *The Yeast Connection Cookbook*).

Get rid of the processed and prepared junk foods, which have hydrogenated or partially hydrogenated fats, as well as those containing food coloring and additives. Replace them with modest amounts of olive, walnut, flax seed, sesame and other unprocessed, unrefined oils. Shop mainly around the outer edges of your super-

175

market. Look for fresh and frozen vegetables, fresh meat, poultry, fish, seafood, eggs, olive oil, pure butter, sardines packaged in sardine oil. I especially recommend organically grown foods, which haven't been chemically contaminated. You'll find these foods in many health food stores and in some supermarkets.

# What You Can Eat During the First Three Weeks

## Foods You Can Eat Freely

### Low carbohydrate vegetables

These vegetables contain lots of fiber and are relatively low in carbohydrates and calories. You can eat them fresh or frozen, cooked or raw.

| | | |
|---|---|---|
| Asparagus | Dandelion | Parsley |
| Beet Greens | Eggplant | Parsnips |
| Broccoli | Endive | Peppers, bell |
| Brussels sprouts | Garlic | Radishes |
| Cabbage | Green pepper | Rutabaga |
| Carrots | Kale | Shallot |
| Cauliflower | Kohlrabi | Snow Peas |
| Celery  Leeks | Lettuce(all varieties) | Soybeans |
| Chard, Swiss | Mustard greens | Spinach |
| Collard greens | Okra | String beans |
| Cucumbers | Onions | Tomatoes |
| Daikon | | Turnips |

### Meat and Eggs

| | | |
|---|---|---|
| Chicken | Salmon | Turkey |
| Mackerel | Beef, lean cuts | Cod |
| Veal | Sardines | Pork,lean cuts |
| Tuna | Lamb | Wild game |

Shrimp, lobster, crab and other seafood
Other fresh or frozen fish

### Nuts, seeds and oils (unprocessed)

| | |
|---|---|
| Almonds | Olive |
| Brazil nuts | Safflower |
| Cashews | Sunflower |
| Filberts | Soy |
| Pecans | Walnut |
| Pumpkin seeds | Corn |

Oils, cold pressed and unrefined
Butter (in moderation)
Flaxseed

## Foods You Can Eat Cautiously

### High Carbohydrate Vegetables

| | |
|---|---|
| Artichoke | Avocado |
| Beans, peas and other legumes | Beets |
| Bonita (white sweet potato) | Breadfruit |
| Potatoes (sweet) | Celery root (celeriac) |
| Winter, acorn or butternut squash | Eggplant |
| Fennel | Whole grains |
| Barley | Corn |
| Kamut | Millet |
| Oats | Rice |
| Spelt | Teff |
| Wheat | |

### Grain alternatives

Amaranth     Buckwheat     Quinoa

### Breads, biscuits and muffins

All breads, biscuits and muffins should be made with baking powder or baking soda as a leavening agent. You'll find recipes and more information in *The Yeast Connection Cookbook*. Do not use yeast unless you pass the yeast challenge as described later.

# Foods You Must Avoid

**Sugar and sugar-containing foods**
Avoid sugar and other quick-acting carbohydrates, including sucrose, fructose, maltose, lactose, glycogen, mannitol, sorbitol, galactose, monosaccharides and polysaccharide. Also avoid honey, molasses, maple syrup, maple sugar, date sugar, and turbinado sugar.
**Packaged and processed foods**
Canned, bottled, boxed and other packaged and processed foods usually contain refined sugar products and other hidden ingredients.
*You'll not only need to avoid these sugar-containing foods the early weeks of your diet, you'll need to avoid them indefinitely.*

## Avoid yeast containing foods the first ten days of your diet.

Here's a list of foods that contain yeast or molds:
**Baked Goods:** Breads, Pastries and other raised baked goods.
**Cheeses:** All cheeses. Moldy cheeses, such as Roquefort, are the worst.
**Condiments:** Sauces and vinegar-containing foods: Mustard, ketchup, Worcestershire, Accent (monosodium glutamate); steak, barbecue, chili, shrimp and soy sauces; pickles, pickled vegetables, relished, green olives, sauerkraut, horseradish, mince meat and tamari. Vinegar and all kinds of vinegar containing foods, such as mayonnaise and salad dressing. (Freshly squeezed lemon juice may be used as a substitute for vinegar in salad dressings prepared with unprocessed vegetable oil).
**Malt products:** Malted milk drinks, cereals and candy. (Malt is sprouted grain that is kiln-dried and used in the preparation of many processed foods and beverages).
**Processed and smoked meats:** Pickled and smoked meats and fish, including bacon, ham, sausages, hot dogs, corned beef, pastrami and picked tongue.
**Edible fungi:** All types of mushrooms, morels and truffles.
**Melons:** Watermelon, honeydew melon and, especially cantaloupe.
**Dried and candied fruits:** Raisins, apricots, dates, prunes, figs, pineapple.

**Leftovers:** Molds grow in leftover food unless it's properly refrigerated. Freezing is better.

After you've avoided yeast containing foods for ten days, you can find out if you are sensitive to yeast, which you can obtain from a health food store. If it doesn't bother you, eat some moldy cheese.

If consuming these yeasty foods triggers symptoms, stay away from them for several weeks. Then you can experiment further.

Truly yeast-free diets are impossible to come by because you'll find yeast and molds on the surfaces of all fruits, vegetables and grains. Once you've found out that you're sensitive to yeast, you'll need to be your own judge as to how much you tolerate food that may contain some yeasts or molds.

During the first three weeks of your diet avoid fruits. The sugar in fruits, although combined with fiber, are more quickly released and may trigger yeast overgrowth. But to see if they bother you, you can do the fruit challenge. Here's how:

Take a small bite of banana. Ten minutes later, eat a second bite. If no reaction occurs in the next hour, eat the whole banana.

If you tolerate the banana without developing symptoms, try strawberries, pineapple or apple the next day. If you show no symptoms following these fruit challenges, chances are you can eat fruit in moderation. *But feel your way along and don't over do it.*

## What You Should and Should Not Drink

**Water:** You should drink eight glasses of water a day. Yet, ordinary tap water may be contaminated with lead, bacteria or parasites.

**Fruit juices:** These popular beverages are a "no no". Most fruit juices, including frozen, bottled or canned, are prepared from fruits that have been allowed to stand in bins, barrels and other containers for periods ranging from an hour on up to several days or weeks. Although juice processors discard fruits that are obviously spoiled by mold, most fruits used for juice contain some level mold.

**Coffee and tea:** These popular beverages, including the health food teas, are prepared from plant products. Although such products are subject to mold contamination, most people seem to tolerate them. To decide, you can experiment. Teas of various kinds, including taheebo (Pau d'Arco) and mathake tea, have been reported to have therapeutic value. If you can't get along without your coffee, limit your intake to one or two cups a day. Drink it plain or sweetened with stevia or liquid saccharin.

**Alcoholic beverages:** Wines, beers and other alcoholic beverages contain high levels of yeast contamination, so if you're allergic to yeast, you'll need to avoid them. You should stay away from alcoholic beverages for another reason: They contain large amounts of quick-acting carbohydrate. If you drink such beverages, you'll be feeding your yeast.

**Diet Drinks:** These beverages possess no nutritional value. More-over, they're usually sweetened with aspartame (Nutrasweet$^{TM}$), which causes adverse reactions in many people. They may also contain caffeine, food coloring, phosphates and other ingredients, which disagree with many individuals. However, since diet drinks do not contain mold, some people with candida related problems may tolerate them. If you drink them, use them sparingly.

# Meals:

The menus listed and illustrated on the next few pages are all *sugar-free* and *yeast-free* and designed to help you answer the always troublesome question, *What can my family and I eat?*

The menus for the early weeks are also fruit-free and contain relatively few grains and high carbohydrate vegetables (such as potatoes, yams and lima beans). Depending on your likes and dislikes, using these general guidelines, you can change these menus to suit your tastes and those of other members of your family.

If you pass "the yeast challenge," you can cautiously add cheeses, mushrooms, and other yeast-containing foods to your diet on a rotated basis. *You should also rotate your other foods, especially during the early weeks and months of your treatment program.* Here's why:

Many, and perhaps most, individuals with yeast-connected health problems are allergic to several (and sometimes many) different foods. The more frequently you eat a particular food, the greater the chances of developing a "hidden" allergy to that food. Such an allergy may contribute to your fatigue, headaches, muscle aches, depression or other symptoms. And strange as it may seem, you may become addicted to the foods that are causing your symptoms, so you crave them.

You can find menus and suggestions that will make carrying out your diet detective work much easier in *The Yeast Connection Cookbook* which I co-authored with Majorie Hunt Jones, R.N. This book contains more than 225 recipes, which will help you with your meal planning.

## Meal Suggestions for the Early Weeks

**Breakfasts:**
-3\4 to 1 cup cooked oatmeal with butter or flaxseed oil and pecans.
-3\4 cup cooked brown rice with filberts, sardines packed in sardine oil and rice cakes.
-Well cooked eggs, 2 strips of crisp bacon and 3\4 cup of cooked grits with butter.
-Oatmeal, pork chops and cashew nuts.
-Brown rice, sardines in sardine oil, rice crackers and filberts.
-Cooked quinoa, baked sweet potato and pecans.

**Lunches:**
-Pork chops with broccoli, sesame/oat crackers, sliced potatoes.
-Beef patty, one cup of string beans, filberts, steamed cauliflower.
-Turkey breast, baked sweet potato.
-Salmon, carrots, rice cakes, turnips, cabbage.
-Vegetable soup (or Progresso TM lentil soup), rice cakes,almonds.
-Tuna fish with lemon and chopped celery; pecans salad with tomato, lettuce, green pepper, cucumber and radish; flaxseed oil and lemon juice dressing; rice cake.

**Suppers:**
-Baked Cornish hen, steamed cabbage, asparagus, salad with lettuce and pecans. Use walnut oil and lime juice dressing.
-Steak (or hamburger patty), eggplant, mixed green salad with cucumbers and green peppers.
-Pork chops or lamb chops, turnip greens, okra, carrot and celery sticks.
-Roast Turkey, baked acorn squash, steamed spinach, grated cabbage, almonds with lemon juice and flax oil dressing.

-Mixed vegetables cooked in microwave, pecans.
-Tuna fish, broccoli, black-eyed peas.

## After the first several weeks of your diet, you can experiment.

### And the chances are you can eat freely
All fresh vegetables.
All fresh fruits (in moderation).
Whole grains (in moderation).
You can continue to consume fish, lean meat, egg, nuts, seeds and oils. And if you pass the yeast challenge test, you can also include some of the yeast containing foods.

### You must continue to avoid
Sugar, maple syrup, honey, corn sugar, date sugar and sugar containing foods: Packaged and processed foods of low nutritional quality that contain sugar and hydrogenated or partially hydrogenated fats and oils.

## Meal Suggestions After the First Few Weeks

### Breakfast
-Ground beef patty, scrambled eggs, grits with butter, apple sauce muffin.
-Pork chop, steamed Brussels sprouts, whole wheat biscuit, grape-fruit.
-Toasted rise cakes with peanut butter, sliced banana, turkey burger.
-Brown rice with butter and chopped almonds, tuna (water packed), fresh pineapple.
-Eggs, well cooked, any style; pancakes made with teff, spelt, kamut; freshly squeezed orange juice.
-Barley cereal with banana and pecans, milk, fish (baked or broiled).
-Hot oatmeal with cashews, milk and fresh or frozen peaches.

### Lunches
-Salmon patty, corn bread boiled cabbage, black eyed peas, sliced

tomatoes, orange.
-Fish cakes, steamed cauliflower, boiled okra, rice cakes, strawberries.
-Tuna salad on lettuce, rice cakes, steamed green beans, boiled Brussels sprouts, fresh pineapple.
-Swiss steak, steamed artichoke, turnip greens, raw carrots, corn bread.
-Chicken salad, rice soup, spinach, rice biscuits, apple.
-Pork chop, lettuce and tomato salad, applesauce muffin, baked banana.
-Meat loaf, barley soup, celery and carrots, whole wheat biscuits, pears.

## Suppers
-Sautéed liver, lima beans, baked acorn squash, sliced tomato, banana oat cake.
-Broiled fish, cabbage & carrot slaw, wax beans, whole wheat popovers, baked banana.
-Broiled lamb chops, steamed cauliflower, steamed broccoli, boiled potatoes, baked apple.
-Rock Cornish hen, steamed carrots and peas, wild rice, rice crackers.
-Roast duck, kale, barley soup, sweet potato, steamed green beans, corn bread.
-Broiled steak, baked potato, lettuce tomato, cucumber salad and freshly squeezed lemon juice and safflower or linseed oil dressing, mixed greens, fresh strawberries.
-Chicken and rice, steamed artichoke, turnip greens, corn bread, pear.

# Shopping Tips

Feature whole foods: Avoid foods labeled "enriched" if you are allergic to yeast.

Use fresh fruits and vegetables. Commercially canned products often contain yeasts and added sugar. Buy fresh organic vegetables when possible.

Since many, and perhaps most canned, packaged and processed foods contain hidden ingredients, including sugar, dextrose and other carbohydrate products, avoid them.

If you must use canned or packaged foods, *read labels carefully.*

If buying frozen vegetables, select those without added ingredients, such as fancy sauces.

Avoid processed, smoked or cured meats, such as salami, wieners, bacon, sausage and hot dogs, since they often contain sugar, spices, yeasts and other additives. Such foods also are loaded with the wrong kind of fat.

Avoid bottled, frozen and canned juices. If you want juice, buy fresh fruit and prepare your own.

Buy nuts from a natural food store where there is a rapid turnover and the nuts are less apt to be rancid or contaminated with molds. Store them in your refrigerator or freezer. Avoid peanuts if you are allergic to yeasts or molds.

All commercial breads, cakes and crackers contain yeast. If you wish yeast-free breads, you'll have to obtain them from a special bakery or bake your own. Word of caution: Many people with yeast related problems react adversely to wheat. So, if you continue to experience symptoms, you may need to avoid breads and similar products. Hain or Chico San or Golden Harvest Rice Cakes contain no sugar or yeast. Most rice cakes contain no sugar.

Use expeller-pressed vegetable oils, such as sunflower, safflower, flaxseed and corn. Flaxseed oil is a superb source of the important Omega 3 essential fatty acids. To make salad dressing, combine the oil with fresh lemon juice to taste.

Buy whole grain (barley, corn, kamut, millet, oats, rice, spelt, teff and wheat) from a natural food store. Grains can be important ingredients of a nutritious breakfast. Barley, rice and other grains can also be used in various ways at other meals. Barley or rice casseroles are especially tasty.

## More Helpful Suggestions

If your health problems are yeast-connected, you may improve...often dramatically...when you stop eating foods that contain significant amounts of cane sugar, beet sugar, corn syrup, fructose, dextrose or honey. Then if you follow other parts of the candida-control program, after two or three months you may find you can consume foods that contain a small amount of sugar.

Yet, if you are allergic to yeast and molds, you may pay for any dietary infraction. And you may not achieve maximum improvement until you avoid all foods that contain yeast and molds. So you may need to stay away from spices, sprouts, condiments and un-frozen leftover foods. (Molds quickly grow on any food that isn't eaten as soon as it's prepared).

Then if you're still experiencing problems, you'll need to carry out food allergy detective work. In so doing, you identify and avoid all foods that cause adverse or allergic reactions. Common offenders include milk, egg, wheat, corn and soy. However, any food can be a troublemaker. Identifying hidden food allergies requires a carefully designed and appropriately executed elimination diet.

Every person differs from every other person. *You are unique*. In following the anti-candida diet, use a trial and error approach. Most of my patients with candida-related illness, as they improve, can follow a less rigid diet, especially if they're following other measures to regain their health. Included are the use of nutritional supplements, exercise, stress reduction and avoiding exposure to environmental chemicals and mold spores.

## Eating Out

If you're like most people, you live "on the run" and eat foods away from home. What's the answer? Do the best you can. And during the early weeks and months of your candida-control program, you may need to do a lot of brown-bagging. And when you eat out, you'll need to make selections carefully, to avoid foods that trigger your symptoms.

## Eggs

Fresh, well cooked (Important because eggs may be contaminated with salmonella bacteria) whole eggs offer many ingredients needed to build and maintain strong health. They contain all eight essential amino acids, the building blocks of high quality protein, and are rich in essential fatty acids (EFAs). These two groups of nutrients are "essential" in diet because they aren't made in the body. Eat eggs hard boiled, poached or scrambled. Don't fry them because when you cook them at high temperatures the fat breaks down and produces harmful substances called trans-fatty acids.

## Vegetables

*These plant foods are good for* you. And there are many you can choose, including cabbage, broccoli, collard greens, soy beans, Brussels sprouts, onions, carrots, tomatoes and others. You should eat five (or more) servings *every* day. Here are some of the reasons why vegetables play a critical important role in promoting optimal health:

-They're loaded with vitamins, minerals, fiber and *complex* carbohydrates.

-They contain *phytochemicals*. There are hundreds of these substances in plant foods. You've probably read or heard about some of them, including genistein in soy beans, flavones in dried beans and indoles and isothiocyanates in broccoli. There are many more, some not yet identified.

-They contain adequate protein.

-Vegetarian diets lessen your chances of developing osteoporosis, heart disease, diabetes and other degenerative diseases, which affect tens of millions of Americans who consume high protein, high fat diets.

Although I included meats in the menus for the early weeks, I urge you to improve the quality of your diet in the months ahead by eating less meat. Here's one reason: *Animal foods are loaded with pesticide residues.* So eat more plant foods, including vegetables, fruits and whole grains. You'll find a comprehensive discussion of the reasons why such diets promote good health in many other publications.

## Sweetened Foods And Beverages
Here's why they cause symptoms:

-When you eat simple sugars, you encourage yeast overgrowth in your digestive tract. A 1993 study in mice showed that the intestinal growth of candida was approximately 200 times greater in mice receiving dextrose than in a group that didn't receive sugar.

-Diets containing large amounts of refined sugar cause your pancreas to put out extra insulin. As a result, rapid up and down fluctuations occur in your blood and brain sugar levels, producing nervousness, weakness, irritability, drowsiness and other symptoms of hypoglycemia.

-When you fill up on sugar laden foods, you're apt to take in insufficient amounts of essential nutrients, including vitamins, minerals. essential fatty acids and phytopharmaceuticals (found in fruits and vegetables). Such nutrients participate in various body enzyme systems and serve as precursors in the manufacture of hormones and neurotransmitters (chemicals your brain requires to function properly).

-You may be allergic to sucrose and other sugars derived from a particular botanical source (Cane, beet, corn or maple).

## Yeast And Mold Containing Foods

Avoiding yeasts and molds in your diet isn't easy. Molds are everywhere, indoors and outdoors. Although dampness and darkness promote mold growth, as do basements and cellars, molds can grow on any food, including fruits, vegetables, nuts, meats, spices and leftovers.

Although heating...even boiling or processing...may kill live molds, mold products may be left behind and this may cause problems for some individuals with candida-related disorders.

Eating a yeast-containing food doesn't make candida organisms multiply. So when you develop symptoms from eating a yeasty food, you develop them because you are allergic to yeast products.

**Leftovers:** Leftover foods provide a rich breeding ground for yeasts and molds. Molds are one of the major microorganisms causing foods to spoil, and all foods spoil. Although refrigeration retards mold growth, even refrigerated foods develop mold contamination. So prepare only as much food as you need and eat it promptly, or freeze leftovers.

**Spices and Condiments:** These dietary ingredients are usually loaded with mold and should be avoided or approached with caution. Limited quantities of salt and juice from freshly squeezed lemon are your safest food flavoring agents. And freshly squeezed lemon juice, plus unprocessed vegetable oil, make a healthy, nutritious salad dressing.

**Dry Cereals:** These cereals, you'll find in the supermarket...even the best of them...have been processed and subjected to high heat. Accordingly, they're much less desirable than hot cereals you prepare at home made from whole grain. Moreover, most of these cereals are loaded with sugar and contain malt and added yeast derived B vitamins. So if you're allergic to yeast, you'll need to avoid them.

If you like dry cereals, you can find some nutritious ones at the health food store. Many of them are organically produced; some of them contain a mixture of grains; and most are fruit sweetened. I especially recommend Health Valley cereals.

If you purchase a dry cereal at your usual grocery store, I suggest sugar-free, yeast-free Shredded Wheat. Other cereals that may be suitable include Cheerios, Puffed Rice, Wheat Chex, Puffed Wheat, Post Toasties, Product 19, and Special K. All have less than 6 percent added sugar. I don't recommend them for the early weeks, but as you improve, you may be able to tolerate these cereals in limited amounts.

## Diversity Or Rotate Your Diet

Even if you aren't able to carry out a carefully designed and executed elimination diet, by rotating your foods you may be able to identify some of that may be disagreeing with you and causing your symptoms.

In rotating your diet, you eat a food only once every four to seven days. For example, in rotating fruits, you'd eat oranges on Monday, bananas on Tuesday, apples on Wednesday and pineapple on Thursday. Then on Friday you could start all over again with oranges (or a related food such as a grapefruit). Do the same thing with other food groups, including meats, vegetables and grains.

## Suggestions For Breakfast And Eating On The Run

Breakfast is your most difficult meal, especially during the early weeks. In the recipe section of *The Yeast Connection Cookbook*, my collaborator and co-author, Marge Jones, commented:

*What can I eat for breakfast? Time and time again I hear this and it is a valid concern for people on a diet to control candida.*

*If you strip breakfast of yeast, you'll eliminate toast, French toast, bagels, sweet rolls, even sourdough bread. If you also omit wheat, milk, corn, sugar, soy and egg, you end up with a gaping void in your menus where breakfast use to be.*

Marge then gives you lots of breakfast suggestions, including muffins, pancakes or flat bread that you can make a few days ahead, package and freeze. Then when you're ready, you can put them in your toaster oven.

Eat these versatile little treasures with your fingers, like dainty pieces of toast, or top them with your favorite filling or bean dip for open-faced mini-sandwiches. They go brown bagging easily and travel well on trips, too.

Marge is a real authority on the non-grain alternatives, amaranth, buckwheat and quinoa. These nutritious foods are high in protein, vitamins, minerals and fiber, as well as rich in complex carbohydrates. They're also useful for people who are sensitive to wheat and corn.

She also tells you how to fix breakfast "pudding". Ingredients in this recipe include foods that you may not consider breakfast foods, such as sweet potatoes and other vegetables. Another suggestion, especially during the diagnostic phase of your diet, is a big bowl of oatmeal with chopped nuts or well-cooked eggs with lean meat.

When eating on the run, plan ahead. Don't wait until you're rushing off to work. Make sure that you can fill your "brown bag" with nutritious foods, including raw vegetables, nuts and rice cakes. You also may get some of the nutritious vegetable based burgers from your health food store.

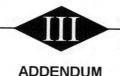

# Elimination Diet

**<u>Major Caution</u>**: Do **<u>NOT</u>** eat any food you already know causes a severe allergy. This diet is to detect foods that you eat frequently but that are **<u>NOT</u>** presently recognized as a possible cause of certain medical, behavior, activity or learning problems.

## MULTIPLE FOOD ELIMINATION DIET, PART 1
How do you do the first part of the diet?

During the first week, most meats, fruits and vegetables can be eaten. (The 'allowed' and 'forbidden' foods are listed below). Keep detailed records in a food diary of **exactly** what is eaten. Most individuals who are going to respond favorably to this diet do so about the 6th or 7th day; others respond as early as the 2nd or, rarely, as late as the 14th day.

If you are better in a week or less, begin Part 2 of the diet on the 8th day. Improvement noted on day 2 may greatly increase by day 7. The object is to see the maximum amount of improvement which can be noted during the first 7 days.

If you want to help your entire family, urge everyone to try the diet at the same time. Typically, **several** family members will note improvement in how they feel or act when this is done.

If you are **not** better within a week, re-check the diet records for the initial week of the diet. Were **only** the allowed foods eaten? If you repeatedly forgot and ate the wrong foods or drank the wrong beverages at school, work or home, the item which was **not** deleted or omitted from the diet may be the culprit. Try Part 1 of the diet again, but this time try much harder to adhere strictly to the diet. It's best to do the diet only one time, but do it right. This fast, inexpensive method of food allergy detection can sometimes provide rapid, safe relief of many chronic medical and behavioral complaints.

Occasionally, a person is worse during Part 1 of the diet. **If this happens, immediately stop the diet.** A frequent cause is that the patient has begun to ingest an excessive amount of an unsuspected offending food or beverage. A child who substitutes apple or grape juice for milk, for example, may act or behave much worse if apple or grape juice is the cause of this child's symptoms. Retry Part 1 of the diet, but stop the suspect food or beverage which you think made you or your child worse.

Rarely, a person who was not helped during the first week will dramatically improve with a more prolonged diet. Continue Part 1 of the diet for two weeks, not one week. If Part 1 of the diet is tried and has not helped by the fourteenth day, this particular diet is probably not the answer for you, your child or your family. The medical problems are not related to foods or are possibly due to other frequently eaten or craved items, i.e. mushrooms, cinnamon, coffee, tea, tobacco, etc., which were not removed from the diet.

**If an infection occurs during the diet, stop the diet until you are well. It is too difficult to interpret the results if it is continued.**

During Part 1 of the diet, the following foods are omitted in all forms: milk and dairy products (yogurt, cheese, ice cream, casein, sodium caseinate, whey), wheat (bread, cake, cookies, baked goods), eggs, corn, sugar, chocolate (cocoa or cola), peas, peanut butter, citrus (orange, lemon, lime, grapefruit), food coloring, food additives and preservatives. No luncheon meats, sausage, ham or bacon are allowed. If there is some question about a specific food, do **not** eat it. Also, exclude any other food or beverage that is craved in excess because such items are frequently unsuspected causes of various medical or emotional problems.

# MULTIPLE ELIMINATION DIET- PART 1
(Read all labels first)

## ALLOWED | ## FORBIDDEN

### CEREALS
Rice - Rice Puffs only
Oats - Oatmeal made with honey
Barley

### CEREALS
Foods containing wheat flour
(most cakes, cookies, bread & baked goods)
Corn, popcorn
Cereal mixtures (Granola)

### FRUITS
Any fresh fruit, except citrus.
Canned (if in their own juice, without artificial color, sugar or preservatives)

### FRUITS
Citrus
(orange, lemon, lime and grapefruit)

### VEGETABLES
Any fresh vegetables,
except corn and peas
French fries (homemade)
Potatoes

### VEGETABLES
Any frozen or canned vegetables
Corn
Peas
Mixed vegetables

### MEATS
Chicken or turkey (non-basted)
Louis Rich ground turkey
Veal or beef
Pork
Lamb
Fish, tuna

### MEATS
Luncheon meats, wieners, bacon
Artificially dyed hamburger/meat
Ham
Dyed salmon, lobster
Breaded meats
Meats with stuffing

### BEVERAGES
Water
Single herb or plain tea & honey
Grape juice, bottled (Welch's)
Frozen apple juice (Lincoln or pure apple)
Pure pineapple juice (no corn or dextrose)

### BEVERAGES
Milk or dairy drink with casein or whey
Fruit beverages except those specified
Kool-Aid
Coffee Rich (yellow dye)
7-Up, Squirt, Teem, cola, Dr. Pepper, ginger ale

### SNACKS
Potato chips (no additives)
Rykrisp crackers and pure honey
Raisins (unsulfured)

### SNACKS
Corn chips (Fritos)
Chocolate/Cocoa
Hard candy, ice cream or sherbet

### MISCELLANEOUS
Pure honey
Homemade vinegar/oil dressing
Sea Salt
Pepper
Pure maple syrup
Homemade soup

### MISCELLANEOUS
Sugar
Bread, cake, cookies (except special recipes)
Eggs, cheese
Dyed (colored) vitamins, pills, mouthwash, toothpaste, medicines, cough syrups, etc,
Jelly or jam, Jell-O
Margarine or diet spreads (dyes and corn)
Peanut butter/peanuts
Sorbitol (corn)

193

# MULTIPLE FOOD ELIMINATION DIET, PART 2
How do you do the second part of the diet?

| | |
|---|---|
| add MILK | on Day 8 |
| add WHEAT | on Day 9 |
| add SUGAR | on Day 10 |
| add EGG | on Day 11 |
| add COCOA | on Day 12 |
| add FOOD COLORING | on Day 13 |
| add CORN | on Day 14 |
| add PRESERVATIVES | on Day 15 |
| add CITRUS | on Day 16 |
| add PEANUT BUTTER | on Day 17 |

During Part 2 of the diet, one food is reintroduced into the diet, in excess, each day. Keep detailed records of how you feel at the beginning and the end of each day, and observe carefully for one hour after a food is tried or eaten again. Start with a teaspoon or ½ cup of the test food item and double the amount eaten every few hours, so that by the end of the day at least a 'normal' amount has been ingested. Do any symptoms suddenly reappear? If there are **no** symptoms during that day, during the night or the next morning before breakfast, the food tested the day before is probably all right and may be eaten whenever desired. If the test food causes symptoms, stop eating it **in all forms** until you can secure the advice of your physician. Do not give yourself another test food until the symptoms for the previous food test have subsided. Usually you will notice that symptoms caused by a food occur within one hour. Symptoms such as canker sores, tight joints, ear fluid, bowel problems and bed wetting (in children) can be caused by a food and tend to cause delayed reactions several hours later.

If symptoms persist, Alka-Seltzer Antacid Formula without aspirin (gold foil) or Alka-Aid can be purchased from the health food store. (Dose is 1 tablet for a 6 year old, 2 tablets for a 12 year old). Don't use if liver or kidney disease is present. The usual allergy medications can be taken, so your symptoms subside quickly. If concerned, check with the doctor.

**REMEMBER:** if one of the listed foods causes a reaction which is not helped by Alka-Seltzer in the gold foil and which lasts over 24 hours, **DO NOT TRY** to check the response to another possible problem food until the reaction has **entirely** subsided.

Watch closely to see what happens each day. One food might cause a stuffy nose, the next, no reaction at all, the next a bellyache. Some reactions occur immediately, others in several hours. **Once again, if a food obviously causes serious symptoms, it should not be tried.**

**NEVER TEST ANY FOOD WITHOUT YOUR DOCTOR'S ADVICE IF IT CAUSED SERIOUS MEDICAL PROBLEMS IN THE PAST. FOR EXAMPLE: IF EGG OR PEANUTS CAUSED SERIOUS THROAT SWELLING OR FISH CAUSED SEVERE ASTHMA, IT IS UNSAFE TO TRY EVEN A SPECK OF THESE FOODS.**

If you are uncertain whether a food causes symptoms or not, discontinue it until the other foods have been checked. Then try the food again at a five day interval, i.e.: Tuesday and Saturday. See if the symptoms recur each time.

If you want to learn even more about what food does when it is eaten again, do the following:

1. Write and draw. Does either change or deteriorate before and twenty minutes after a food is eaten?

2. Take your pulse. If it increases by 20 to 40 points after eating a particular food, once again your body could be warning about some food sensitivity.

3. Use a Pocket Peak Flow Meter if you have asthma. Use this before and 20 minutes after each food. If the reading on the gauge fall 15%, or 50 or so points, that food or beverage could be the cause of wheezing.

## SPECIFIC DETAILS OF PART 2 OF DIET:

**Day 8: The day you add milk**: have plenty of milk, cottage cheese and whipped cream sweetened with **pure** maple syrup or honey. Not butter, margarine or yellow cheese unless you are absolutely certain they contain NO yellow dyes.

**Day 9: The day you add wheat**: add Triscuits or pure wheat cereal. If you had trouble from milk, be sure NOT to have milk products. Use Italian bread or kosher bread because these should not contain milk (casein or whey), **but always read labels to be sure**. You can bake if you'd like, but you must not use eggs or sugar. Remember, you can eat no dairy products or drink any milk if these seemed to cause medical problems. If milk caused no problem, milk products can be eaten.

**Day 10: The day you add sugar**: give your child sugar cubes to eat and add granulated sugar to the allowed foods. If milk or wheat caused trouble, they must be avoided or you can't tell if sugar is tolerated. Many children react within one hour after 4-8 sugar cubes.

**Day 11: The day you add egg**: have eggs in usual forms, cooked or as eggnog. Have custard. Remember, no wheat, milk or sugar can be consumed of any of these caused problems. Be sure to skip this food challenge if you already know egg is a problem.

**Day 12: The day you add cocoa**: have dark chocolate with water, cocoa (pure Hershey's cocoa powder) and honey or pure maple syrup. No candy bars are allowed because most contain milk and corn. Remember, no milk, wheat, sugar, dyes or eggs are allowed if any of these caused symptoms.

**Day 13: The day you add food coloring**: have Jell-O, jelly or artificially colored fruit beverages (soda pop, Kool-Aid), popsicles or cereal. Try to have lots of yellow, purple and red items because you may react to only one of these colors. Remember to avoid milk, wheat, cola or sugar in all forms if any of these were a problem. If sugar caused symptoms, use honey or pure maple syrup, as a sweetener or add food coloring to plain pure gelatin. If milk, wheat or sugar were tolerated, they may be eaten.

**Day 14: The day you add corn**: Have corn, corn meal, corn flakes, and plain popcorn. The latter can be made with salt. If milk, wheat, sugar, dyes, eggs or chocolate cause trouble, you can't have them on the same day you have corn. If you do and symptoms are worse you won't be able to tell which is at fault. Do not use butter on popcorn if you have a milk sensitivity.

**Day 15: The day you add preservatives**: have foods which contain any preservatives and food additives. Read every label. In particular, eat luncheon meat, bologna, hot dogs, bread, baked goods, or soups which contain many preservatives and additives.

**Day 16: The day you add citrus**: have large amounts of lemon, lime, grapefruit or orange as fresh fruit, or in juice. Avoid artificial dyes if food colors were a problem.

**Day 17: The day you add peanut butter**: have lots of peanut butter or peanuts. Test for this only if it's a favorite food. Use Rykrisp if no wheat is allowed. Use pure peanut butter without additives (Smuckers).

## Special Tips For The Multiple Elimination Diet

The allowed foods can be selected, combined and eaten in any quantity. If you are a bit suspicious, start with a tiny amount and increase it during the day if no symptoms are revealed.

For a beverage, you can mix the allowed fruits in the blender with spring water and honey or pure maple syrup. Use these on cereal to replace milk. Use carbonated water to create soda pop.

Your usual medications can be taken during the diet. If you begin to improve, you may find that certain medicines such as antihistamines are needed less often by the end of the first week. Try to use only white pills or colorless liquids. Most liquid medications contain corn, sugar, artificial flavors, and artificial dyes which can cause symptoms.

Once you determine which foods cause specific symptoms, you must discuss the problem with your physician. Some foods cannot be omitted for indefinite periods of time if proper nutrition is to be maintained.

**Do not try the diet if you have an infection or are receiving an antibiotic which contains dyes, sugar, flavoring or corn.**

Although symptoms from a single food vary, food sensitivities are often evident in several family members. For this reason, urge the entire family to do the diet. One child might develop headaches, another a stuffy nose, a third, hyperactivity, and another child might wet the bed. The same food, i.e., milk, can be a problem for several generations of a family. For this reason, make cooking easier by placing the entire family on the diet. A fringe benefit may be that you relieve some 'emotional or learn-to-live-with-it' type health problems caused by certain foods or beverages in several family members.

If you have children and your child refuses the diet, try offering a reward. Promise a gala party if there is no cheating and if it is obvious that the child is truly trying very hard to cooperate in every way. The party should take place AFTER both parts of the diet are completed. At that time, give your child the foods which caused the symptoms providing they were not severe or incapacitating. This will be a double check confirming the effect of these foods on your child. Alka-Aid (available at health food stores) will prevent or stop reactions in many children in 10-15 minutes depending upon whether it is given **before** or **after** a food is eaten.

If you or your child has asthma, add the test food back into the diet with extreme care. It is possible that an unsuspected food could precipitate a sudden severe asthma attack. Have asthma medications on hand during Part 2 of the diet and use the Pocket Peak Flow Meter to help find out exactly what is causing any wheezing. If you are concerned or your asthma has ever been severe or frightening, check carefully with you doctor before trying this diet.

If you or your child are worse during the first 2 to 3 days after the diet, this could just be 'normal' withdrawal symptoms (i.e., nausea, headache, irritability). These usually subside by the fourth day. If you or your child are worse by the 5th or 6th day, suspect whatever you substituted for milk or whatever you are eating in excess while you are on the diet (i.e., potatoes).

If you are routinely worse (impatient, angry, tired, irritable, headachy, hyperactive) **before** meals, think about hypoglycemia or low blood sugar. If this is your problem, merely eating a small protein snack every hour or two all day might make you stay on a more even keel and feel much better.

# INDEX

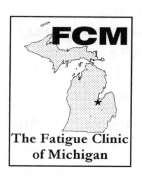

The Fatigue Clinic
of Michigan

To contact
# The Fatigue Clinic of Michigan

Phone (810) 230-8677
Fax (810) 230-7855
or
Write
The Fatigue Center of Michigan
G3494 Beecher Road
Flint, MI 48532

# ORDER FORM

FAX ORDERS              810-230-7855

TELEPHONE ORDERS        810-230-8677

MAIL ORDERS

> Vitality Press, Inc.
> G3494 Beecher Road
> Flint, MI 48532

Please Send Me _____ Copies
### of America Exhausted

☐ Please send me Information on the
### Fatigue Clinic of Michigan Newsletter

| | |
|---|---|
| NAME | |
| ADDRESS | |
| CITY | |
| STATE | ZIP |
| PHONE | |

**SHIPPING: $4.00 for first book, $1.00 each additional book.**

**SALES TAX: Michigan residents please add sales tax.**

Copies @ 14.95 each = _____

Shipping _____

Tax _____

Total _____

**Make Checks or Money Orders Payable to Vitality Press**